BOOK 4

FROM NEURONS TO BEHAVIOUR

This publication forms part of an Open University course SD226 *Biological Psychology: Exploring the Brain*. The complete list of texts which make up this course can be found on the back cover. Details of this and other Open University courses can be obtained from the Course Information and Advice Centre, PO Box 724, The Open University, Milton Keynes MK7 6ZS, United Kingdom: tel. +44 (0)1908 653231, e-mail general-enquiries@open.ac.uk

Alternatively, you may visit the Open University website at http://www.open.ac.uk where you can learn more about the wide range of courses and packs offered at all levels by The Open University.

To purchase a selection of Open University course materials visit the webshop at www.ouw.co.uk, or contact Open University Worldwide, Michael Young Building, Walton Hall, Milton Keynes MK7 6AA, United Kingdom for a brochure: tel. +44 (0)1908 858785; fax +44 (0)1908 858787; e-mail ouwenq@open.ac.uk

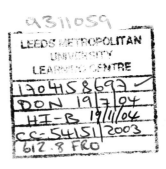

The Open University
Walton Hall, Milton Keynes
MK7 6AA

First published 2004

Copyright © 2004 The Open University

Edited, designed and typeset by The Open University.

Printed and bound in the United Kingdom by the Alden Group, Oxford.

ISBN 0 7492 6626 0

1.1

SD226 COURSE TEAM

Course Team Chair

Miranda Dyson

Academic Editor

Heather McLannahan

Course Managers

Alastair Ewing
Tracy Finnegan

Course Team Assistant

Yvonne Royals

Authors

Saroj Datta
Ian Lyon
Bundy Mackintosh
Heather McLannahan
Kerry Murphy
Peter Naish
Daniel Nettle
Ignacio Romero
Frederick Toates
Terry Whatson

Multimedia

Sue Dugher
Spencer Harben
Will Rawes
Brian Richardson

Other Contributors

Duncan Banks
Mike Stewart

Consultant

Jose Julio Rodriguez Arellano

Course Assessor

Philip Winn (University of St Andrews)

Editors

Gerry Bearman
Rebecca Graham
Gillian Riley
Pamela Wardell

Graphic Design

Steve Best
Sarah Hofton
Pam Owen

Picture Researchers

Lydia K. Eaton
Deana Plummer

Indexer

Jane Henley

Cover image: *Vision at End of Day* by Mark Rothko (National Gallery of Art, Washington)

Contents

NEURONAL COMMUNICATIONS

1.1 Introduction

In Book 1 you were introduced to the concept that the nervous system is a dynamic community of interconnected and interdependent cells that function together to determine how our bodies (and minds) interact with, and respond to, the external and internal world. Of the many cell types that make a brain, it is the neuron, and the synaptic connections it makes with other neurons (to form the neural network), which represent the communications hub of the nervous system. Each day our brains perform countless computations, processing a wealth of information through the action of interconnected neural networks. An appreciation of how these networks function will aid your understanding of how the brain works, and how brain function can be affected by damage and disease, and be influenced by the administration of drugs; chemicals such as cocaine, levodopa, Ecstasy and nicotine. As mentioned earlier, neurons use electrical signals (action potentials) and synaptic transmission to communicate, often at considerable speed over relatively large distances. How neurons work together to achieve this is discussed in the following sections.

1.2 Electricity and the neuron

To understand how a neuron uses electricity to communicate, it is helpful to consider how the electricity is generated and stored. The electrical energy of a cell is created by an unequal distribution of electrically charged atoms and molecules (called ions) on either side of the plasma membrane. (You were first introduced to ions in Book 1, Section 2.4.1.) Ions can be either negatively or positively charged. An example of a positively charged ion is sodium, written as Na^+. (Na is the chemical symbol for sodium and the plus sign indicates that it carries a single positive charge.) Another example of a positively charged ion is calcium, Ca^{2+}. (In this case calcium carries two positive charges.) An example of a negatively charged ion is chloride, and it is written as Cl^-.

Figure 1.1 shows the distribution of ions between the inside and the outside of a typical neuron. You will notice that there are many more sodium ions contained in the extracellular fluid (outside the cells) and many more potassium ions in the intracellular fluid (inside the cells), and it is this unequal distribution of these charged potassium and sodium ions across the plasma membrane that provides the electrical energy used by neurons to communicate. This unequal distribution of molecules across the membrane is a common feature of most cells.

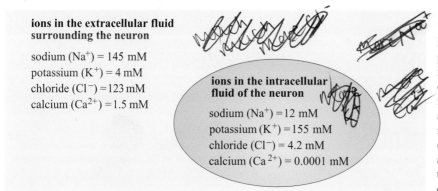

ions in the extracellular fluid surrounding the neuron

sodium (Na^+) = 145 mM
potassium (K^+) = 4 mM
chloride (Cl^-) = 123 mM
calcium (Ca^{2+}) = 1.5 mM

ions in the intracellular fluid of the neuron

sodium (Na^+) = 12 mM
potassium (K^+) = 155 mM
chloride (Cl^-) = 4.2 mM
calcium (Ca^{2+}) = 0.0001 mM

Figure 1.1 The concentrations of sodium, potassium, chloride and calcium ions found inside a neuron and in the surrounding extracellular fluid are shown. In addition to the ions shown, the neuron also contains an abundance of large, negatively charged, organic molecules. (The concentration units are in mM (millimoles). However, you do not need to worry about the units – all you need to appreciate is that the larger the value, the greater the concentration.)

This ionic distribution results in a voltage (also called the *potential difference*) across the plasma membrane. We can measure the potential difference using a voltmeter connected to a microelectrode inserted into a neuron (see Figure 1.2). A typical neuron has a potential difference of about −70 millivolts (mV); that is, the inside of the cell is 70 mV more negative than the outside of the cell. This potential difference across the plasma membrane is called the **membrane potential**. It is important, at this point, to appreciate that the cell shown in Figure 1.2 is in a resting state; or in other words, the cell is quiescent (it has a stable and steady membrane potential); it is not involved in electrical communication with other cells. In the resting state the membrane potential recorded is called the *resting* membrane potential; so we can say that the cell illustrated in Figure 1.2 has a resting membrane potential of −70 mV. A membrane potential is not an exclusive property of electrically excitable cells such as neurons and muscle cells. Other cells, such as glia and red blood cells for example, also have resting membrane potentials and these too are a function of the distribution of ions across their plasma membranes. In the case of these cells, the energy stored in the form of the membrane potential is used to drive other processes, such as the transport of other molecules into and out of the cell.

To understand how a neuron maintains its resting membrane potential, we must first consider the forces at play on either side of the membrane, and for the purposes of this discussion, we will only consider the role of sodium and potassium ions.

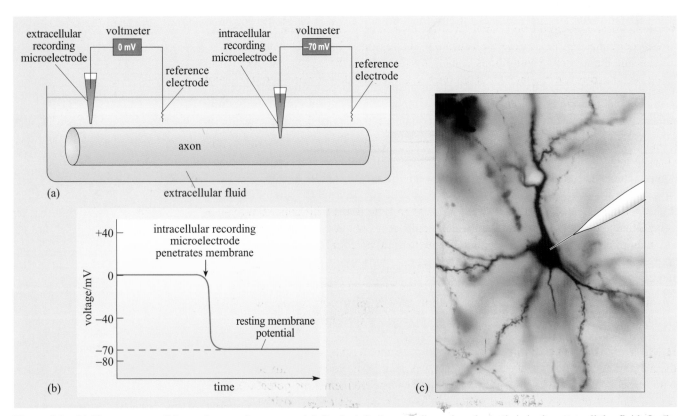

Figure 1.2   (a) Measurement of the resting membrane potential. On the left, the recording microelectrode is in the extracellular fluid. On the right, when the microelectrode has penetrated the axon and entered the intracellular fluid the voltmeter displays the membrane resting potential (−70 mV). (b) The change in potential as the microelectrode penetrates (impales) the membrane. In this case, the cell is at its resting membrane potential. (c) A photograph of a cortical pyramidal neuron in a slice of brain tissue taken using a light microscope. For illustrative purposes an intracellular recording microelectrode has been superimposed.

The resting membrane potential tells us something about the amount of electrical energy stored by the cell. A general property of molecules in solution, in our case ions, is that they have a continuous random motion. As a result, dissolved substances, such as ions, tend to 'spread out' from a region of high concentration to a region of low concentration until they are evenly distributed – the molecules are said to move down a **concentration gradient**. The process whereby substances in a liquid (or gas) attain uniform distribution is called *diffusion*. Unless something prevents the passage of the molecules, diffusion ultimately produces a uniform mixture of molecules; the concentration of each component is the same throughout the medium. The plasma membrane can be thought of as a barrier restricting the diffusion of ions from a region of high concentration to a region of low concentration.

◆ As we saw earlier in Figure 1.1, there is an unequal distribution of sodium and potassium ions on either side of the plasma membrane. Ions, like all small molecules are constantly moving. What do you think would happen to the distribution of these ions if they could diffuse freely through the plasma membrane?

◆ Over time, the ions would redistribute evenly across the membrane. The ions would diffuse from areas of high concentration to areas of low concentration; they would flow down their concentration gradient.

◆ In which direction would the potassium and sodium ions flow?

◆ Potassium ions would flow down their concentration gradient, from the region of higher concentration, inside the neuron, to the region of lower concentration, outside the neuron. Sodium ions would also flow down their concentration gradient, from the region of higher concentration, outside the neuron, to the region of lower concentration, inside the neuron.

From the above we can infer that (i), at rest, the membrane is relatively impermeable to both sodium and potassium ions, and (ii), if the membrane was freely permeable to charged molecules, then potassium ions would leave the cell and sodium ions would enter.

◆ If sodium and potassium ions were allowed to flow down their concentration gradients so that eventually they were evenly distributed across the plasma membrane – what would happen to the membrane potential?

◆ The membrane potential arises because of the unequal distribution of ions across it. Perturbations of this distribution will affect the membrane potential – a cell in which all the ions were evenly distributed across its plasma membrane would have a membrane potential of zero mV.

In addition to the concentration gradient across the membrane, another force at play is the membrane potential itself. If you recall, the inside of the cell is negatively charged with respect to the extracellular fluid (the cell has negative membrane potential); this can be thought of as an **electrical gradient**. As a result, ions with a positive charge will be attracted by the negative charge of the cell.

Two factors contribute to the generation of the resting membrane potential. The first factor is that there is an abundance of large *negatively* charged organic molecules (often referred to as organic anions), the majority being proteins, trapped within the

cell. The second factor is that the resting membrane is slightly permeable (leaky) to potassium ions. The leakage of positively charged potassium ions from the cell, as the ions flow down their concentration gradient, increases the overall electrical negativity of the intracellular compartment and thus helps to maintain the negative membrane potential. Indeed, when in its resting state, the resting membrane potential of a neuron is almost entirely attributable to the distribution of potassium ions on either side of the plasma membrane.

◆ Describe the factors that contribute to the resting membrane potential.

◆ The resting membrane potential is due to the leakage of positively charged potassium ions out of the cell (down their concentration gradient) and the presence of organic anions inside the cell.

It was mentioned earlier that the distribution of potassium ions across the membrane largely determines the membrane potential. However, this relationship starts to fail as the membrane potential approaches or becomes more negative than the resting membrane potential. At more negative membrane potentials, the ability to accurately predict the membrane potential from the distribution of potassium ions starts to fail. The reason for this is that whilst the membrane is relatively permeable to potassium ions, it is also slightly permeable to sodium ions, so at more negative potentials sodium ions are drawn into the cell by the increase in the electrical gradient as the cell becomes more negative.

◆ If the leakage of potassium out of and the entry of sodium into the cell remained unchecked, what would happen to the membrane potential?

◆ The cell would gradually lose the ability to maintain a negative membrane potential. Eventually, the cell would have a membrane potential of zero mV.

So, how is the unequal distribution of potassium and sodium ions maintained? This is achieved by the presence of a specialized protein that sits in the plasma membrane and 'pumps' sodium ions out of and potassium ions into the cell. This pump, called the **sodium–potassium pump**, uses cellular energy derived from a special molecule, ATP, to drive the pumping process. (ATP is the energy molecule used to drive most living processes.) At rest, the sodium–potassium pump consumes 40% of all cell energy (or in other words, 40% of the energy in the food that you eat is used to maintain the distribution of ions across the cell membranes). The importance of the sodium–potassium pump for maintaining the distribution of sodium and potassium ions across the membrane is easily demonstrated by the drug ouabain; a compound that selectively inhibits the pump. Cells exposed to ouabain gradually lose their ability to maintain a negative resting membrane potential and, if the drug is not removed, the cells will eventually perish. Figure 1.3 shows a schematic diagram of the sodium–potassium pump in action.

◆ Look at Figure 1.3. Note that for every two potassium ions pumped into the cell, three sodium ions are expelled. What significance will this have in terms of the membrane potential?

◆ Each time the pump exchanges sodium for potassium, a net positive charge is exported from the cell. The action of the pump will add to the negativity of the membrane potential.

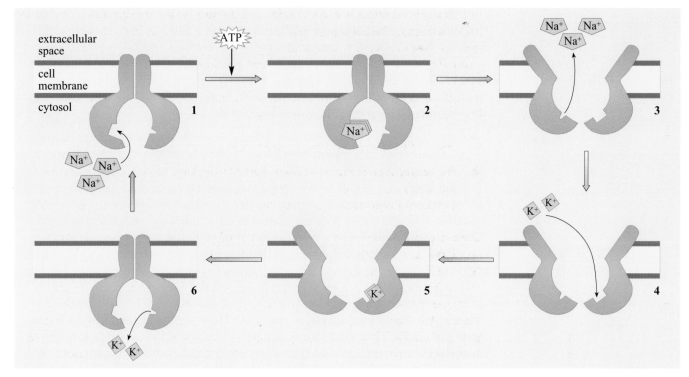

Figure 1.3 A schematic diagram showing the sodium–potassium pump. Note that the pump extrudes three sodium ions for every two potassium ions taken up by the cell.

However, the pump does not deplete the cell of sodium ions because other cellular processes draw sodium into the cell. Details of these other processes are beyond the scope of this course.

1.3 Electricity in action

1.3.1 Ion channels in action

So far, our discussion has concentrated on how cells are capable of generating and maintaining a voltage across their plasma membrane – to be a 'living' battery. We will now focus on how this electrical energy is used to generate electrical signals. However, first it is necessary to think about how ions cross plasma membranes. In Book 1, Section 2.4.1 you were introduced to the concept of the cell membrane as a fluid mosaic; a sea of lipid molecules with a host of floating proteins (Book 1, Figure 2.12). Imagine a membrane made entirely of lipid molecules; such a membrane would be impervious to the passage of charged molecules – ions would be unable to pass through it. In order for an ion to pass through our imaginary lipid membrane, a hole or pore is required. In the case of the neuronal membrane the holes are made by specialized proteins. These proteins form structures called **ion channels** (sometimes called protein channels) that span the plasma membrane, allowing ions to pass through them (an example of a protein channel is shown in Figure 2.12 of Book 1). Indeed, we have already mentioned the role that potassium ions play in the generation of the resting membrane potential – this crucial leak of potassium ions is through a special type of ion channel, a potassium ion-selective channel called the **passive potassium channel**.

◆   How do you think you could show that passive potassium channels contribute to the resting membrane potential?

◆   You could use a chemical to block the channel and record the change in membrane potential.

◆   What would happen to the membrane potential?

◆   Blocking the potassium channels would prevent the leak of positively charged potassium ions from the inside of the cell to the extracellular fluid. As a consequence, the membrane potential would be more positive than if the leakage had continued.

Evolution has produced a diverse and complex array of ion channels – in terms of their ion selectivity, how they are opened or closed, and the responses they evoke. This diversity is amply demonstrated by the way that ion channels work together, in an exquisitely orchestrated manner, to produce the action potential.

The action potential is the main neuronal output signal (often referred to as the *nerve impulse*). As you will learn in the next section it is ideally suited for this role.

Figure 1.4a shows a typical action potential illustrating the key steps in the action potential profile. (For the moment do not concern yourself how the action potential was elicited; we will return to this subject shortly.) The action potential is a very brief but dramatic change in the membrane potential – the change can be as much as 100 mV. The action potential consists of a **depolarization** phase (the membrane potential becomes less negative) briefly achieving a membrane potential of +20 mV or more, followed by a phase of **repolarization** (when the membrane potential returns (repolarizes) to the resting membrane potential) and a short period of **hyperpolarization** (when the membrane potential becomes more negative than the resting membrane potential).

Perhaps the simplest way of illustrating the events underlying the action potential is first to describe the changes that occur in terms of the plasma membrane permeabilities for sodium and potassium ions. As we have already said, most cells have resting membrane potentials in the range of −60 to −80 mV. At these resting potentials, the cells are said to be quiescent – they are not actively generating action potentials and their membrane permeabilities for potassium and sodium ions are low (just the leakiness mentioned earlier). Should a small part of the cell be made less

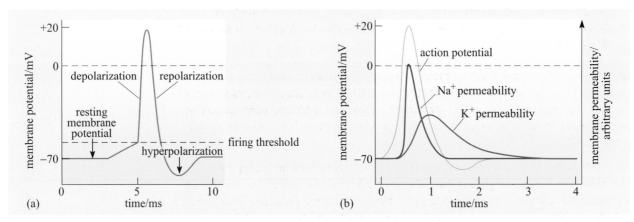

Figure 1.4   (a) A typical action potential. (b) A graph showing an action potential with the membrane permeability changes for sodium and potassium superimposed. Note how the change in potassium is delayed with respect to the change in sodium permeability.

negative, i.e. an event occurs that produces a local depolarization in the cell (we will learn more about these events later), and if the depolarization is sufficiently large, the cell will generate an action potential. Typically, the membrane potential at which an action potential is initiated is about −55 mV, i.e. about 15 mV more positive than the resting membrane potential. At this potential, called the **firing threshold** (or threshold potential) a small part of the membrane suddenly becomes permeable to sodium ions which then enter the cell driven by both their chemical and electrical gradients. The entry of positively charged sodium ions rapidly makes the membrane potential less negative, indeed, for a brief moment the plasma membrane potential becomes positive, reaching a level of about +20 to +30 mV (i.e. 90 to 100 mV more positive than the resting membrane potential, see Figure 1.4). At the very peak of the action potential, during the phase of maximum depolarization, the membrane permeability to sodium ions suddenly and dramatically decreases; effectively switching off the flow of sodium ions into the cell.

Important features of the action potential are that it is rapid, transient and local. Thus a cell can generate an output signal and then rapidly recover so it is ready to generate a further signal, if required. The way the cell quickly recovers its membrane potential is to lose positively charged ions. This is achieved by a change in the membrane permeability to potassium ions – to rapidly restore the resting membrane potential, the membrane now becomes permeable to potassium ions. These ions leave the cell, driven by the potassium concentration gradient, and in doing so, remove positive charge from the intracellular fluid, making the cell more negative – in other words, the plasma membrane repolarizes. Indeed, for a brief period, the cell becomes more negative (hyperpolarized) than the resting potential – the role of this hyperpolarizing phase will be discussed in the next section. However, before we move on, it is important to note that during the depolarizing and repolarizing phases of the action potential, only a small fraction of the available sodium and potassium ions actually move across the membrane. The changes in membrane potential are localized: the whole cell is not depolarized, just a tiny portion of it – ions in the immediate vicinity are affected but, as only a small area of membrane is involved at any one time, only a few ions actually move.

◆ What is the advantage gained by the cell if only a small number of ions participate in the generation of an action potential?

◆ The advantage of this arrangement is that the underlying voltage or electrical energy stored in the cell is not depleted (the 'battery' is not run down or discharged by a single action potential) so that a cell can continue to generate action potentials.

So, at one level, we can think of the action potential as an orchestrated duet between the membrane permeabilities for sodium and potassium ions, as shown in Figure 1.4b. Here we can see that the rapid increase in membrane permeability to sodium precedes the change in potassium permeability, which is also slower and longer lasting.

How can a membrane alter its permeability to ions to generate an action potential? The answer is fairly straight forward; the permeabilities for sodium and potassium are mediated separately by specialized ion channels in the membrane. The action potential is initiated by the opening of **voltage-gated sodium channels** – channels that are sensitive to the voltage across the membrane, i.e. they respond to changes in the membrane potential. At the resting membrane potential, these channels are

closed, but when the membrane is sufficiently depolarized, the channels open; it is the voltage at which these channels open that determines the firing threshold. The channels remain open until the cell is depolarized to about +20 mV, at which point they close and enter a period of inactivation – *inactivated sodium channels can no longer contribute to the generation of actions potentials.* At this point, a second set of voltage-gated channels, the potassium channels, come in to play. These channels are also sensitive to the membrane potential and open in response to the depolarization of the cell to +20 mV. Their opening is *delayed* with respect to the initiation of the action potential and consequently, these channels are known as the **delayed voltage-gated potassium channels** (not to be confused with the passive potassium channels discussed earlier). These delayed potassium channels allow potassium to leave the cell, rapidly repolarizing the membrane. The movement of potassium through the open channels briefly makes the cell more negative than the resting membrane potential; it is said to be hyperpolarized. This period of hyperpolarization is an important feature of the action potential as it plays a role in the reversal of sodium channel inactivation. An inactivated voltage-gated sodium channel is unresponsive and it remains in this state until the channel experiences a period of membrane hyperpolarization, at which point, the inactivation is removed and the channel is free to contribute to future action potentials. The voltage-dependent processes of activation and inactivation confer two important characteristics upon the action potential.

- The first is that the action potential is an *all-or-nothing* event. Once voltage-gated sodium channels are activated, an action potential will ensue – in other words, once the firing threshold has been achieved, the cell will produce an action potential.

- The second is that, once inactivated, the channels can no longer open – these channels remain in this dormant inactivated state until they experience a period of hyperpolarization; channels which do not experience a period of hyperpolarization will eventually return to their resting state, but do so slowly.

As long as the channels remain inactivated, the cell cannot produce another action potential – the cell is said to be in a **refractory** state. In other words, the rate at which a cell can generate action potentials is determined by the duration of the refractory period. (There is a section on ion channels in the multimedia package *Exploring the Brain.*)

The voltage-gated sodium channel is an important target for the treatment of several neurological conditions, including epilepsy. Neurons can generate action potentials at amazing rates, as many as a hundred or more per second. (The maximum firing rate for each cell is determined by the type of ion channels present on that cell.) During an epileptic episode, many neurons fire action potentials in synchrony with each other, with ever increasing frequency; eventually this abnormal pattern of activity dominates the brain resulting in a seizure or fit. By placing electrodes on the scalp of a patient it is possible to record that patient's brain activity – this type of recording is called an electroencephalogram (EEG; see Book 3, Section 2.4.1). Figure 1.5 shows a recording made from a patient who suffers from epilepsy. At the beginning of the recording the patient has a normal pattern of brain activity. However, this suddenly and dramatically changes as the patient enters the seizure state: the EEG shows an increase in electrical activity and a characteristic pattern of peaks indicating the synchronous firing of a large number of neurons. One of the most successful drugs

used in the prevention of epileptic seizures is phenytoin, a drug that reduces the synchronous firing of neurons and decreases the rate of action potential firing by impairing the efficiency of the sodium channel (effectively increasing the duration of the refractory period). Whilst this drug can act on all neurons, it only produces its effect in those neurons involved in the generation of trains of action potentials, such as those involved in the abnormal brain activity seen in epilepsy.

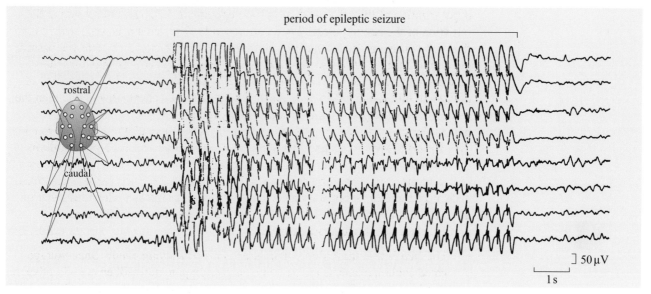

Figure 1.5 The inset on the left shows the location of electrodes on the scalp of a patient suffering from epilepsy. The traces correspond to the activity recorded from different pairs of electrodes as indicated. The traces show electrical activity from several brain areas and show the synchronous firing of a large number of neurons during an epileptic seizure.

Another drug commonly used in medicine and dentistry, this time as a local anaesthetic, is lidocaine (lignocaine); a compound that blocks the pore of the sodium channel. In particular, this drug prevents the generation of action potentials in axons involved in nociception, so that the patient is unable to 'feel' pain arising from the treated region.

Before we consider how, once generated, an action potential is capable of transmitting information, you should be aware that the above description of the resting membrane potential and the action potential is far from being a comprehensive one. We have made several simplifications to facilitate understanding, and in doing so we may have given the impression that neurons sit happily at their resting membrane potential unless provoked into generating an action potential. Whilst this is true for a large variety of neurons found in the nervous system, there are some notable exceptions. Some cells fire action potentials spontaneously (you will learn more about these cells in a later section of this chapter). These cells contain a multitude of different ion channels that together generate a rhythmic 'pace-maker' potential which repeatedly bring the cells to their firing threshold. As we will learn later, these cells play an important role in regulating the properties of neural networks. An example of a rhythmically firing neuron, in this case a cell which releases the neurotransmitter dopamine, is shown in Figure 1.22b.

1.3.2 The generation of the action potential: overview

Now, you can think of the action potential in terms of a small number of steps. Depolarization, if large enough to reach the threshold, opens voltage-gated sodium channels and an action potential occurs: the membrane potential moves from the resting potential of about -70 mV towards a potential of about $+20$ mV (Figure 1.4). The sodium channels close after less than a millisecond, and the membrane voltage returns to the resting potential as a result of the delayed voltage-gated potassium channels opening.

◆ What features of the delayed voltage-gated potassium channels contribute to the period of membrane hyperpolarization in the last phase of an action potential?

◆ (a) The channels open later than the sodium channels as the membrane potential rises from -70 mV to zero.

(b) The delayed voltage-gated potassium ion channels stay open for a relatively long period after sodium ions have stopped flowing.

As a first approximation, such a sequence of events helps us understand what happens when an action potential is generated. The 'real life' action potential is more complicated. But the description given so far is adequate for our current needs. It has highlighted the process of channel opening and closure as vital factors in determining the state of a neuron. As well as contributing to an understanding of the action potential, an awareness of the effects of channel opening and closure can give insight into the ways that drugs and other chemicals can exert their influence upon the nervous system – by opening, closing or blocking channels for specific ion types.

1.3.3 Propagation of the action potential

Once generated, where does the action potential go? You will recall that most neurons found in the brain consist of a cell body with a dendritic tree and an axon (see Book 1, Figure 2.18). Within a neuron, the highest density of sodium channels is found at the axon hillock, the transitional structure between the cell body and the axon. Depolarizing events (we will discuss the origins of these later) that occur within the dendrites and cell body spread along the plasma membrane. If these events bring the membrane at the axon hillock to its firing threshold, an action potential is generated. The action potential then 'rushes off' at considerable speed down the axon. How is this achieved?

Figure 1.6 shows a 'snapshot' of an axon with an action potential 'travelling' along it. The action potential can be visualized as invading the axon in two waves, an initial depolarizing wave (due to the opening of the voltage-gated sodium channels) closely followed by a repolarizing/hyperpolarizing wave (due to the opening of the delayed voltage-gated potassium channels). As a piece of membrane depolarizes during the passage of the action potential, the sodium channels in the membrane adjacent to it 'sense' the depolarization and in turn are also recruited (i.e. opened). This process is repeated again and again, enabling the propagation of the action potential along the length of the axon. Another important feature of the action potential is that it propagates away from the site of initiation – in other words, it will travel away from the axon hillock along the axon. The action potential also travels from its site of

initiation at the axon hillock back into the cell body and dendrites – a process known as back-propagation. (The role of back-propagated action potentials is complex and poorly understood, however, they are believed to be involved in regulating the properties of the dendrite.) As the action potential passes down the axon, the axonal membrane becomes refractory, thus preventing the back-propagation of the action potential.

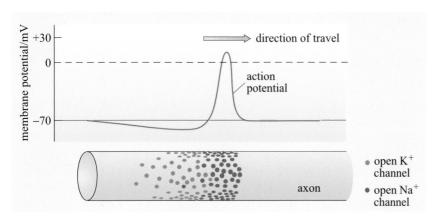

Figure 1.6 A 'snapshot' of an axon with an action potential travelling from left to right. (*top*) The action potential. (*bottom*) The wave of sodium (red) and potassium (purple) channels opening that give rise to the action potential indicated on the axon.

As mentioned earlier, the action potential is the output signal used by the brain to pass information from neuron to neuron. In the case of the muscles in your foot, the cell bodies of the neurons controlling them are located over a metre away in the spinal cord! Clearly, the speed at which an action potential passes along the axon (the conduction speed; also referred to as the rate of conduction or conduction velocity) is a crucial factor in the efficient processing and transfer of information.

Not all axons conduct action potentials at the same speed, and this is illustrated in Figure 1.7. So far we have only considered the action potential recorded in a single neuron or axon. Using a different type of electrode (an extracellular electrode) it is possible to record action potentials in a nerve containing several hundred axons. (Remember axons in nerves are also referred to as nerve fibres.) By applying an electric shock to the nerve, it is possible to evoke an action potential in most of the axons in the nerve. If the electric stimulus is applied at a known distance from the recording electrode, then as the evoked action potentials pass beneath the recording electrode their activity and the time taken for them to travel to the recording site is recorded. Because the distance travelled and the time taken is known, it is possible to calculate the speed of conduction. In Figure 1.7b the recorded response is shown, consisting of three humps or peaks: A, B and C. These correspond loosely to three groups of action potentials passing beneath the recording electrode at different times. These peaks arise because the axons in the nerve have different conduction speeds. To distinguish this type of potential from that recorded in a single axon, we refer to it as a **compound action potential**. The main factor that determines the speed of conduction is the presence or absence of a myelin sheath. (You first came across myelin in Book 1, Section 2.4.4.) In addition to this, the diameter of the fibre also has an effect, such that speed is proportional to the diameter (the greater the diameter, the faster the speed of conduction). The properties of the fibres that contributed to the compound action potential shown in Figure 1.7 are listed in Table 1.1. (A similar table is presented in Book 1, Table 2.3.)

Figure 1.7 (a) A sketch of a simple experimental set-up to evoke and record a compound action potential in a nerve. Because the distance between the stimulation and recording sites can be measured, the speed of conduction can be easily calculated. (b) The compound action potential recorded from a nerve found in the leg. At time zero on the time axis, the nerve was stimulated and the resulting potential has typically three peaks, labelled A, B and C. Expansion of peak A (see insert, note also the expanded time scale) reveals three distinct peaks termed alpha (α), beta (β) and gamma (γ) – corresponding to the main populations of neurons that give rise to peak A.

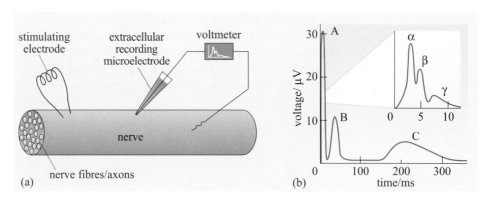

◆ Examine the properties of the fibre types listed in Table 1.1. What is the relationship between diameter and speed of conduction?

◆ The slowest conducting axons are the C fibres, these have the smallest axonal diameter, but they are also unmyelinated, so given the above it is not at all surprising that they have the lowest speed. However, the A and B fibres are all myelinated – for these myelinated fibres, it is the axonal diameter which determines their relative speed of conduction.

Table 1.1   Classification of nerve fibres that give rise to the compound action potential.

Fibre type	Fibre diameter/µm	Speed/m s^{-1}
Aα (also Ia)	8–20	50–120 (myelinated)
Aβ (also II)	5–12	30–70 (myelinated)
Aγ	2–8	10–50 (myelinated)
Aδ	1–5	3–30 (myelinated)
B	1–3	3–15 (myelinated)
C	<1	<2 (unmyelinated)

Each labelled peak in the compound action potential shown in Figure 1.7b corresponds to the fibre types listed above. A and B type fibres are myelinated whilst the C class fibres are not.

How can the presence of a myelin sheath increase conduction speed? To answer this we must first consider the nature of the myelin sheath. Myelin is produced by specialized glial cells (oligodendrocytes in the brain and Schwann cells in the peripheral nervous system – you were introduced to them in Book 1, Section 2.4.4). These cells wrap the axon with a spiral of myelin layers; an example of this is shown in Figure 1.8. There is a small gap between the successive myelin sheaths. The gap is termed a node of Ranvier. Nodes of Ranvier occur every 0.5–2 mm and are about 1–2 µm in length. The myelin sheaths and nodes of Ranvier play a crucial role in the propagation of an action potential, as described below.

Despite their small size, the membrane patches exposed at the nodes of Ranvier have a very high density of voltage-gated sodium channels. In an unmyelinated axon, the action potential propagates along the axon as each successive patch of membrane is depolarized to the firing threshold. In a myelinated axon, the myelin sheath alters the electrical properties of the axon, so instead of smoothly invading each successive patch of membrane, the action potential now jumps from one node of Ranvier to the next; greatly increasing the conduction speed compared with unmyelinated axons of the same diameter. Damage to the myelin sheath or degeneration of the myelin-producing cells can dramatically slow or stop the conduction of action potentials.

$1000\,\mu\text{m} = 1\,\text{mm}$

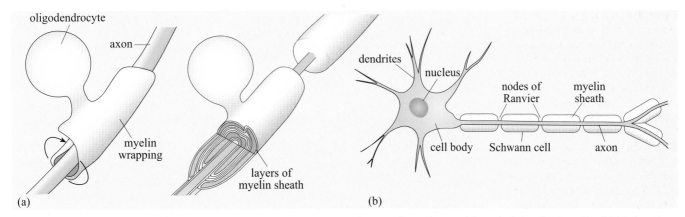

Figure 1.8 (a) A specialized glial cell, called an oligodendrocyte coats the axonal membrane with a spiral sheath of myelin. (b) Nodes of Ranvier are gaps between successive myelin sheaths.

Several diseases of the nervous system, most notably multiple sclerosis, involve the loss of myelin (see Book 1, Figure 2.29). Demyelination is often a complication associated with viral infections such as chicken pox and measles and produces a host of symptoms ranging from muscle weakness to epileptic seizures. Fortunately, demyelination associated with viral infections is usually transitory and patients normally make a full recovery.

Summary of Sections 1.1 to 1.3

The electrical properties of neurons result from the difference in the concentration of ions, particularly sodium and potassium ions, on either side of the plasma membrane. The plasma membrane is a physical barrier to the flow and exchange of ions between the cell and surrounding extracellular fluid. Specialized proteins that form ion channels, span the plasma membrane, providing a route by which ions can pass through the membrane.

The resting membrane potential of a neuron, that is, when it is not transmitting action potentials, is about $-70\,\text{mV}$. This resting potential is maintained in part by the activity of the sodium–potassium pump. The pump is a specialized protein that uses cellular energy (ATP) to pump three sodium ions out of the cell for every two potassium ions pumped into the cell. The exchange of three potassium ions for two sodium ions means that for each cycle of the pump a net positive charge is removed from the cell, thus contributing to the negativity of the membrane potential.

The action potential is a sudden reversal of the resting membrane potential. Action potentials arise due to the ability of neurons to change their membrane ion permeability rapidly. If the axon membrane is depolarized and if this depolarization exceeds the threshold value, an action potential results. Action potentials operate on the all-or-nothing principle, that is, whatever the size of the applied stimulus, as long as it depolarizes the membrane beyond the threshold value (about $-55\,\text{mV}$), exactly the same size of action potential results.

The refractory period follows an action potential. It means that, under normal physiological conditions, an action potential passes along an axon in one direction only.

Axons may be myelinated or unmyelinated. In unmyelinated axons, the action potential travels smoothly along the axon. In myelinated axons, the action potential jumps from one node of Ranvier to the next. For a given diameter of axon, the action potential travels faster along a myelinated axon than along an unmyelinated axon.

1.4   Communication between neurons

1.4.1   Introduction

Thus far we have restricted our discussion to the transfer of information, from axon hillock to axon terminal, in the form of action potentials, within a single neuron. We now consider how neurons communicate with one another in a neural network.

The point of contact between any two neurons is the synapse. The average neuron, by means of its axon terminals, forms about 1000 synaptic connections and it receives even more, perhaps 10 000 connections. Since the human brain contains at least 10^{11} neurons, this means that about 10^{14} synapses are formed. Thus, there are more synapses in one human brain than there are stars in our galaxy! Despite this vast number of connections, information transfer at synapses (synaptic transmission) throughout the nervous system makes use of only two basic mechanisms: chemical transmission and electrical transmission. Before discussing the role and function of chemical synapses (the numbers for synaptic connections mentioned above only relate to chemical synapses), we will first briefly consider electrical transmission.

1.4.2   Electrical synapses: instantaneous communication

Electrical synapses, unlike chemical synapses, provide a means for instantaneous signal transmission between cells and populations of neurons, and until very recently, it was believed that they were of little physiological significance in mammalian brains. (You were introduced to electrical synapses in Book 1, Figure 2.25b.)

Electrical synapses are commonly found in invertebrate animals where they allow the rapid conduction of action potentials and electrical signals from neuron to neuron – allowing groups of neurons to function as a single unit. Ions pass through special protein channels called **gap junctions** between two neurons (Figures 1.9 and 1.10). All gap junction channels consist of a pair of cylinders, one in the presynaptic neuron and the other in the postsynaptic neuron. They meet in the gap between the two cell membranes, forming a channel that connects the cytoplasm of the two cells – in other words, the gap junctions represent a 'direct' physical channel between adjoined cells. Each cylinder is called a connexon and is made up of six identical protein subunits called connexins. The connexins constitute a large family of proteins that differ widely in terms of their sensitivity to modulatory signals and other stimuli such as acidity or levels of chemically reactive molecules that can alter the permeability of the channels. Another important feature of electrical synapses is that, in contrast to chemical synapses which are uni-directional (chemical signals pass in one direction only), electrical synapses are bi-directional – electrical signals can pass in either direction. Figure 1.10 shows the passage of an electrical signal through an electrical synapse.

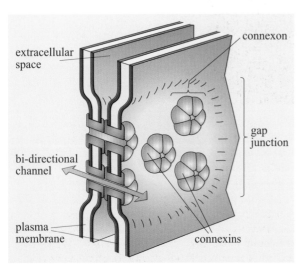

Figure 1.9   A schematic representation of a gap junction – the electrical synapse.

In the laboratory it is possible to demonstrate the existence of gap junctions in mammalian brain tissue by the use of low molecular weight dye molecules that pass

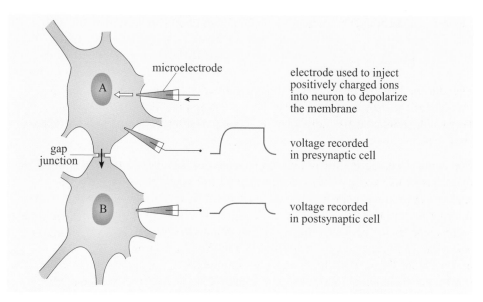

Figure 1.10 Electrical transmission between two electrically coupled neurons. Injection of depolarizing ions into cell A produces a voltage change in cell A that is immediately transferred to cell B via the gap junction. Note that the voltage recorded in cell B is smaller than that seen in cell A. This is because the voltage decays as it spreads passively away from the site of origin (in this case, cell A). The voltage decays as a function of distance from the site of origin – this is explained further in Section 1.5.1 – unlike an action potential which does not decay and is propagated by the sequential opening of sodium channels as it spreads along the axon.

readily through gap junction channels. In the experiment illustrated in Figure 1.11, a hippocampal neuron is filled with a fluorescent dye introduced into the cell using a glass micropipette (Figure 1.11a). The dye rapidly fills the cell body before diffusing into the dendrites and the axon (Figure 1.11b). Within 11 minutes a second neuron also begins to fluoresce (Figure 1.11c). Because the fluorescence is a property of the dye and not the cell, the only way that this second cell can fluoresce is if it too has taken up the dye; and the only route for the dye to pass from cell to cell is via a gap junction. Further examination of the dye-coupled cells shown in Figure 1.11 revealed that the gap junction that allowed the dye to pass between them was located at a point where the axons of both cells briefly came in contact with each other.

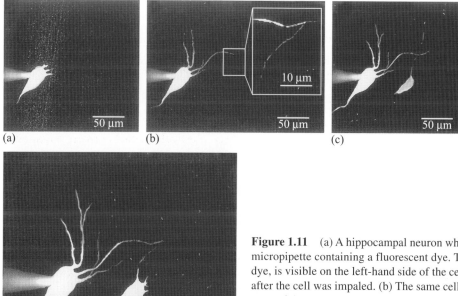

Figure 1.11 (a) A hippocampal neuron which has been impaled by a glass micropipette containing a fluorescent dye. The micropipette, containing the fluorescent dye, is visible on the left-hand side of the cell body. The image was taken 30 seconds after the cell was impaled. (b) The same cell 8 minutes afterwards. The dendrites and axon of the cell are now clearly labelled with the dye. The insert shows the axon of the impaled cell making a physical connection with an axon of a second cell; dye can be seen filling the second axon as it enters the cell via a gap junction made between the two axons. (The scale bar in this insert is 10 μm.) (c) and (d) The same two cells 11 and 17 minutes respectively after being impaled. (The scale bar in all panels, except the insert, is 50 μm.)

The role of electrical synapses in the mammalian brain is only now being addressed. In the retina of the eye, for example, they are involved in the local integration of electrical activity between ensembles of retinal cells. Elsewhere in the brain they are involved in the generation of high-frequency electrical oscillations, similar to those seen during an epileptic seizure. Whilst the function of these gap junction oscillations remains a mystery, it has been proposed that in the cortex and hippocampus they may be implicated in cognitive processing, sensory perception and certain forms of distributed memory formation.

Behavioural testing of animals, in which connexins have been genetically altered so that they are no longer capable of generating these oscillations, is currently underway. This should provide insight into the role of connexins in cognitive and motor function. Current data suggest that the role of gap junctions is to facilitate instantaneous electrical rhythmicity in populations of neurons, if not whole brain structures. It has even been speculated that ultra-high frequency oscillations represent the 'mind' itself! However, despite this speculation, little is currently known about the function of electrical synapses in the human brain, but they do represent a novel and promising site for the development of new therapeutic strategies in the treatment of brain disorders. In the next section we will consider the role of chemical synapses.

1.4.3 Chemical synapses: jumping the gap

Whilst the contribution made by electrical synapses to brain function is only now being investigated, the role that chemical synapses play in processing and initiating brain activity is well documented. Indeed, our current understanding of the brain and how neural networks work is almost entirely dependent on our knowledge of information transfer at chemical synapses. Unlike electrical synapses, where the electrical signal can pass directly from one cell to another, the chemical synapse has to overcome a considerable barrier to the flow of information – a physical divide (a 'gap') that separates the two communicating cells. For the moment, let's consider an axon to be a wire through which the action potential flows; a means of conducting information rapidly over short or long distances in the body. In the nervous system, the axon will make a connection with another neuron, at a specialized structure called a synapse (a chemical synapse). Figure 1.12 shows some examples of the types of chemical synapses found in the brain (also see Book 1, Section 2.4.3). Figure 1.13 shows that the synapse consists of two elements, the presynaptic terminal (also know as the axon terminal or the presynaptic bouton) formed by the axon, and the postsynaptic membrane of the receiving cell. The plasma membranes of the presynaptic terminal and the postsynaptic cell do not make direct contact, instead, they are separated by the synaptic cleft, a small gap of about 20 nm. (Remember 1 nm = 10^{-9} m.) This gap prevents the action potential passing directly from the axon terminal to the postsynaptic neuron. In order for the presynaptic cell to pass on information to the postsynaptic cell, the action potential is converted into a different sort of signal which travels across the synaptic cleft and then generates a response in the postsynaptic neuron. The presynaptic cell achieves this by transforming the action potential (an electrical signal) into a chemical signal that is capable of traversing the synaptic cleft.

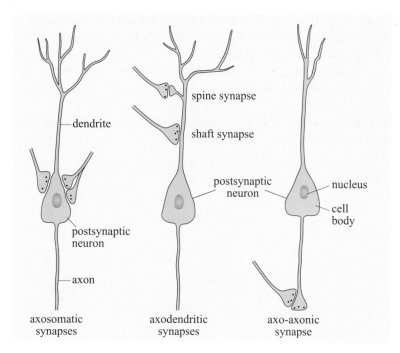

Figure 1.12 Some examples of synaptic connections. Synaptic contact can occur on the cell body, the dendrites, or the axon of the postsynaptic cell. The names of the various kinds of synapses – axosomatic, axodendrtic and axo-axonic – identify the contacting regions between the presynaptic and postsynaptic neurons (the presynaptic element is identified first). Note that axodendritic synapses can occur on either the main shaft of a dendrite branch or on a specialized input structure, the spine.

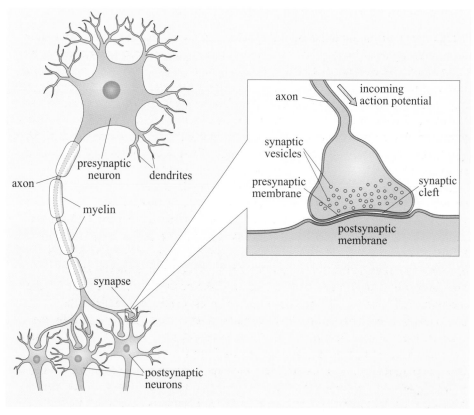

Figure 1.13 Schematic structure of a synapse. Note the presence of synaptic vesicles in the presynaptic terminal. (Remember, not all axons are myelinated in vertebrates.)

◆ Look again at Figure 1.13, what can you see in the presynaptic terminal that is not present at the postsynaptic site?

◆ The presynaptic terminal contains vesicles which are absent at the postsynaptic site.

The presynaptic vesicles are balloon-like structures made from a bilipid membrane (similar in structure to the plasma membrane) that are filled with chemical signalling molecules. The arrival of the action potential at the axon terminal causes some of these vesicles to fuse with the presynaptic cell membrane, releasing their contents into the synaptic cleft (an example of exocytosis; Book 1, Section 2.4.1). The chemical signal then diffuses across the cleft where it binds to specialized proteins on the postsynaptic membrane called receptors. (You were first introduced to receptors in Book 1, Section 2.4.1.) The chemical signal is said to transmit information across the synaptic cleft, so these signalling chemicals are called neurotransmitters (first mentioned in Book 1, Section 1.3.2) and the act of transmission is termed **neurotransmission**. An important feature of neurotransmission is that it is uni-directional; that is, information in the form of vesicular release of neurotransmitter passes from the presynaptic cell to the postsynaptic cell but not in the other direction (i.e. not from postsynaptic to presynaptic cell).

◆   What mechanism ensures that neurotransmission in uni-directional?

◆   Chemical neurotransmission requires the vesicular release of neurotransmitter. Because only the presynaptic site possesses vesicles, neurotransmission can only commence from the presynaptic terminal, hence the uni-directional nature of synaptic neurotransmission – the postsynaptic cell is not equipped to release neurotransmitter into the synaptic cleft.

The arrival of the action potential at the axon terminal initiates the release of the neurotransmitter by activating voltage-gated ion channels found in the presynaptic terminal membrane. These channels are permeable to calcium ions and are normally closed at the resting membrane potential, but open upon depolarization. Arrival of the action potential at the axon terminal briefly causes these channels to open.

◆   Look at Figure 1.1. In which direction will the calcium ions travel when the calcium voltage-gated channels on the membrane of the presynaptic terminal are open?

◆   Calcium will enter the presynaptic terminal of the neuron, flowing down both its concentration and electrical gradients.

The increase in calcium concentration in the presynaptic terminal activates a series of presynaptic proteins which act together to bring about the fusion of synaptic vesicles with the presynaptic membrane and thereby the release of neurotransmitter. The membrane of the synaptic vesicle is then recycled within the terminal to form new vesicles. Figure 1.14 illustrates the key events involved in neurotransmitter release.

At this point of the discussion it is important to appreciate that the majority of neurons normally release only one type of neurotransmitter at their axon terminals, though in some cases, a neuron might have two or more different neurotransmitters in different vesicles. Indeed, there is now evidence to suggest that different neurotransmitters can be localized to different axon terminals of the same neuron. However, for this discussion, we will assume, unless stated otherwise, that a neuron releases the same neurotransmitter at all of its terminals. At this stage in our discussion it is helpful to appreciate that molecules which serve as neurotransmitters come from a variety of sources and synthesizing pathways; indeed, some often have other biological roles in addition to their function as a neurotransmitter, for example, the amino acid glutamate is used as a building block in the synthesis of proteins, as well as being a neurotransmitter.

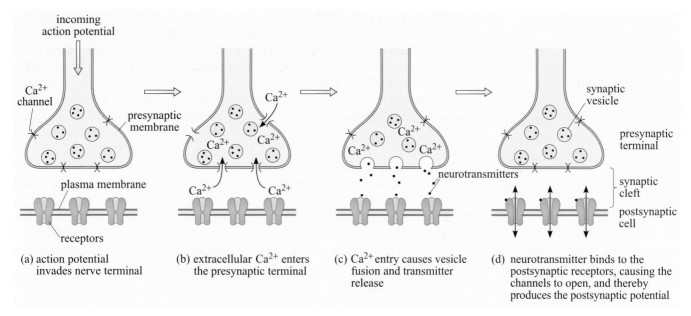

Figure 1.14 Synaptic transmission at chemical synapses involves several steps. (a) An action potential invades the terminal of a presynaptic axon causing calcium voltage-gated channels to open (b). (c) The entry of calcium into the terminal triggers the vesicles containing neurotransmitter to fuse with the cell membrane and release their contents into the synaptic cleft. (d) The released neurotransmitter molecules then diffuse across the synaptic cleft and bind to specific receptors on the postsynaptic membrane. These receptors cause ion channels to open which produce the postsynaptic potential.

Once released from the presynaptic terminal, the neurotransmitter rapidly diffuses across the synaptic cleft and binds to the receptors on the postsynaptic membrane. A given neurotransmitter will bind only to receptors that have a specific binding site for it. One can think of the receptor as being the *lock* and the neurotransmitter as being the *key* with which to open or activate the receptor; in order for the receptor to function, the key must first fit the lock! Neurotransmitters can be thought of as *skeleton keys*, as a given neurotransmitter can bind to several types of receptor, greatly adding to the diversity of responses that can be initiated by a single neurotransmitter. For example, the neurotransmitter acetylcholine acts on one type of receptor found on skeletal muscle (the nicotinic receptor) which triggers muscle contraction and on a completely different type on the heart (the muscarinic receptor) which slows heart rate.

1.4.4   From chemical to electrical signals: re-igniting the spark

Whilst the neurotransmitter provides the means of 'jumping the gap', it is the receptors that re-kindle the electrical response in the postsynaptic cell. Receptors involved in the initiation of electrical activity fall into one of two families that are distinguished by their mode of action. Some receptor proteins are themselves ion channels which open when a neurotransmitter (e.g. glutamate) binds to them. These are called **directly gated ion channels**. Other receptors are not ion channels, but are proteins that, upon the binding of the neurotransmitter (e.g. dopamine), regulate the activity of other proteins and the production of intracellular signalling molecules, called **second messengers** (in this scenario, the neurotransmitter can be thought of as the *first messenger*), which act directly or indirectly to open or close ion channels known as **indirectly gated ion channels**. The direct and indirect regulation of ion channels by neurotransmitters has important implications in terms of the speed of

channel opening and the number of channels activated (see Figure 1.15). Direct activation is fast and generally restricted to the synapse. Indirect activation allows for amplification of the signal, with the result that it can be distributed over a larger portion of the cell; activation of one receptor can lead to the production of a million or so second messenger molecules which in turn can then modify the function of a large number of ion channels or other proteins. Because of the need to generate a second messenger molecule to activate these channels, they are activated more slowly than are directly gated ones. In addition, other intracellular proteins such as enzymes are also activated. The cascade of protein activation and regulation initiated by second messengers often produces prolonged changes and the generation of intracellular messenger molecules that can be further modified by the postsynaptic cell. You will learn later (in Book 5, Chapter 1) that the entry of calcium into cells via directly gated ion channels that are permeable to calcium ions (or voltage-dependent calcium channels that are activated by depolarization) can also activate signalling cascades to generate intracellular messengers that can have far-reaching effects within the cell.

◆ What other presynaptic example of a cellular mechanism/cascade, activated by the entry of calcium, have you already come across?

◆ The entry of calcium into the presynaptic terminal triggers the fusion of vesicles to the presynaptic plasma membrane and the release of neurotransmitter (Figure 1.14).

The binding of the neurotransmitter to the receptor site on an ion channel causes the channel to open; to change its shape so it forms a channel pore through which certain ions can pass. Like the sodium and potassium voltage-dependent ion channels that give rise to the action potential, neurotransmitter-gated channels are also selective for particular ions. This selectivity is very important as it gives rise to one of two types of electrical response in the postsynaptic cell: excitatory or inhibitory. In terms of our understanding of the action of neurotransmitters in this course, all that we need to know is whether the outcome of neurotransmitter activity is excitation or inhibition of the postsynaptic cell.

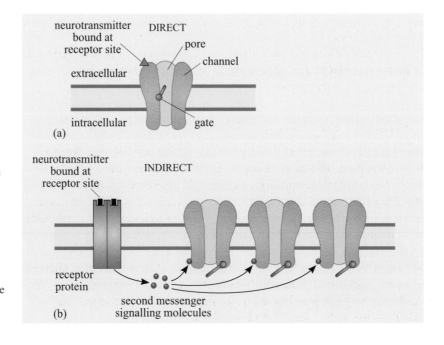

Figure 1.15 Neurotransmission. (a) Directly gated ion channels which give rise to 'fast' synaptic potentials possess both the receptor binding site and the channel, forming a single protein complex. (b) Indirectly gated ion channels give rise to 'slow' synaptic potentials. The binding of neurotransmitter to the receptor protein initiates the production of second messenger molecules (the amplification step) which regulates the opening (or closing) of multiple ion channel protein complexes.

What makes a synaptic connection an excitatory or inhibitory one? The distinguishing feature here is the type of electrical response produced in the postsynaptic cell. An excitatory neurotransmitter, such as glutamate, opens ion channels that depolarize the postsynaptic neuron – because this brings the neuron closer to the firing threshold for an action potential, the effect is said to be 'excitatory' and the electrical response is called the **excitatory postsynaptic potential (EPSP)**. Conversely, an inhibitory response, the **inhibitory postsynaptic potential (IPSP)**, such as that initiated by the inhibitory neurotransmitter GABA (γ-aminobutyric acid), will tend to hyperpolarize the postsynaptic membrane, making it more negative and so reducing the likelihood of generating an action potential. Examples of an EPSP and IPSP are shown in Figure 1.16. See Box 1.1 for more information about amino acids used as neurotransmitters in the nervous system.

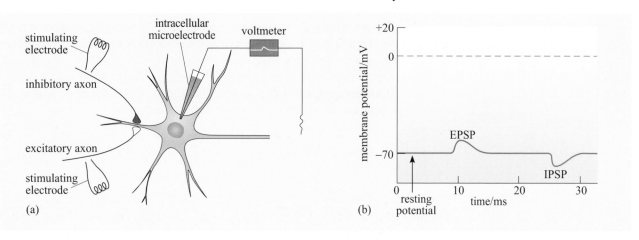

Figure 1.16 (a) An intracellular recording electrode is used to record an EPSP and an IPSP evoked by stimulation of an excitatory input and then an inhibitory input respectively. (b) The EPSP and IPSP recorded in the cell shown in (a).

In terms of the underlying ionic changes at the membrane, neurotransmitter-gated ion channels (both directly and indirectly gated channels) that are excitatory are permeable to sodium and/or calcium ions whilst those that are inhibitory are permeable to potassium or chloride ions.

◆ How do sodium and calcium ions give rise to an EPSP? (Look again at Figure 1.1.)

◆ The entry of positively charged sodium and/or calcium ions into the postsynaptic cell depolarizes it, generating an EPSP. Both ions flow down their respective concentration and electrical gradients.

◆ How do chloride and potassium ions give rise to an IPSP?

◆ Negatively charged chloride ions enter the postsynaptic cell, flowing down their concentration gradient. The entry of negatively charged ions adds to the overall negativity of the postsynaptic cell, generating an IPSP. Potassium ions behave differently. These ions also flow down their concentration gradient, but instead of entering the cell, they leave, removing positive charge and thereby hyperpolarize the postsynaptic cell.

Some neurotransmitters such at glutamate are always excitatory, whereas others such as acetylcholine or dopamine can have either excitatory or inhibitory effects, depending on the type of receptor located at the postsynaptic membrane. The neurotransmitter GABA on the other hand is always inhibitory.

A key feature of neurotransmission is that it is rapid. Whilst the synaptic cleft represents a physical barrier preventing the flow of electrical current from the presynaptic terminal to the postsynaptic cell, the time taken for a neurotransmitter to be released and then evoke an electrical response in the postsynaptic cell is very short; the delay between the arrival of an action potential at the presynaptic terminal and the start of an EPSP is approximately 0.5 ms, this period is called the **synaptic delay**. Another characteristic of neurotransmission is that it is transient. This is due to two processes. First, a relatively small amount of neurotransmitter is released (because the presynaptic action potential is short-lived and the calcium channels that initiate neurotransmitter release at the presynaptic terminal are only transiently activated). Second, the neurotransmitter is rapidly removed from the synaptic cleft or inactivated. There are two basic mechanisms by which a neurotransmitter is removed or inactivated: degradation and removal. Acetylcholine, for example, is inactivated by enzymatic degradation that occurs within the synaptic cleft and at the postsynaptic membrane (the enzyme involved here is acetycholinesterase), whereas glutamate is removed by the action of special 'transporter' proteins in the plasma membrane of the postsynaptic and presynaptic cells (and also other adjacent cells, including glia) that transport it into the cytosol. The glutamate taken up in the presynaptic terminal is then recycled, allowing it to be reused many times. The glutamate taken up by the postsynaptic cell and surrounding glia has a different fate. Here it is converted into the the biologically inert amino acid, glutamine, before being transported out of the cell into the extracellular fluid. (You were introduced to amino acids in Book 3, Section 1.3.) The glutamine is then taken up by the presynaptic terminal where it is converted back into glutmate and repackaged into the synaptic vesicles for future use.

◆ Why is it important that the glutamate removed from the presynaptic cleft by the postsynaptic cell and glia is converted into a biologically inert compound before being recycled?

◆ Glutamate is an excitatory neurotransmitter. The conversion of glutamate to glutamine in the postsynaptic cell and glia allows the converted molecule to be returned to the presynaptic terminal in a manner that does not result in the non-specific activation of glutamate receptors.

The diffusion of neurotransmitter away from the synapses also contributes to the transitory nature of the synaptic potential. In some cases, particularly for certain hormones (hormones were introduced in Book 1, Section 1.3.3), the receptor is *internalized* after activation – it is removed from the plasma membrane and transported into the intracellular compartment of the cell. Depending on the hormone (or neurotransmitter) involved, internalization either switches off the receptor or is the first step in a complex intracellular signalling pathway, a process that often results in gene activation.

Receptors have been distinguished experimentally by the chemical (pharmacological) substances to which they bind and which affect the synapse by occupying either the receptor site or channel pore. Such substances are termed **agonist** and **antagonists**. Agonists are substances which *mimic* the effect of the natural neurotransmitter molecule on the receptor whereas antagonists *inhibit* the action of the natural neurotransmitter. These compounds, together with other drugs that affect the synthesis of neurotransmitters, their removal or inactivation, are used in the study of brain function and the treatment of a host of medical disorders. As

this course progresses you will be introduced to some of these drugs; compounds such as cocaine, nicotine and levodopa. By the end of this course you will begin to understand how these drugs can affect brain function and behaviour.

◆ Can you suggest a compound found in tobacco smoke that might be an agonist?

◆ Tobacco smoking is addictive – this is because tobacco contains an agonist called nicotine, a compound that activates a class of receptors called nicotinic receptors, mentioned in Section 1.4.3. (These belong to the acetylcholine family of receptors – further details can be found in Box 1.2, in Section 1.6.3.)

Smokers find it difficult to give-up their habit – when they try to stop they develop an intense 'craving' to smoke, this is because their nicotinic receptors are not being sufficiently stimulated and the craving, a sign of withdrawal, continues until their next 'fix'. One method commonly used to overcome an addiction to nicotine and smoking is to substitute tobacco with an alternative source of nicotine – commonly, a skin patch that delivers a measured dose of nicotine to the body (the nicotine patch). By gradually decreasing the amount of nicotine in the patch it is possible, over time, to reduce the body's dependence on nicotine, eventually overcoming the addiction.

Box 1.1   Some neurotransmitters

The brain utilizes a host of different chemicals as neurotransmitters. Some of these chemicals, such as acetylcholine are used exclusively as neurotransmitters whereas others, such as the amino acid glutamate have other functions in addition to the role of neurotransmitter. This variety is also reflected in the way neurotransmitters are produced and the methods used to inactivate them once released.

Amino acids

There are a number of amino acids used in the central nervous system. Amongst these is the inhibitory neurotransmitter GABA – a neurotransmitter which is present in all areas of the central nervous system and is mainly found in inhibitory interneurons. A small number of GABAergic neurons are not interneurons, but instead send axonal projections to other brain regions; examples of such cells are the medium spiny neurons of the striatum and the Purkinje neurons of the cerebellum. Following release from the presynaptic terminals GABA is inactivated by reuptake systems; specialized proteins located in the plasma membrane called uptake carriers, that remove GABA from the synaptic cleft. GABAergic neurons can be identified by their ability to accumulate radiolabelled GABA. They can also be identified by the presence of the GABA synthesizing enzyme, glutamate decarboxylase (GAD).

GABA receptors have been identified as important sites for the treatment of several brain conditions such as sleep disorders, anxiety and epilepsy.

Drugs which are thought to act by modifying GABAergic synaptic neurotransmission include benzodiazepines, barbiturates and the anticonvulsant, Valproate.

In the spinal cord, another amino acid, glycine, is used as a neurotransmitter by inhibitory interneurons (see Figure 1.24). Strychnine, a drug used as a rat and bird poison, is a potent antagonist at the glycine receptor. Because strychnine impairs the action of spinal cord inhibitory interneurons to modulate the output of the motor neurons, strychnine poisoning leads to heightened spinal reflexes, eventually causing convulsions characterized by the contraction of most skeletal muscles, followed by complete relaxation. Death usually occurs due to breathing difficulties

Glutamate and aspartate excite virtually all neurons in the brain and spinal cord. Upon release from a glutamatergic terminal, glutamate is inactivated by reuptake into the presynaptic and postsynaptic neurons. Glial cells also possess glutamate reuptake carriers. Here glutamate is converted into another amino acid, glutamine (which does not act as a neurotransmitter), before being released into the extracellular space where it is taken up by the

presynaptic neuron to be converted back into glutamate ready for vesicular packaging and release as described in the text.

Glutamate acts on many different types of receptor. One type, called the N-methyl-D-aspartate receptor (or NMDA receptor) is a neurotransmitter-gated ion channel that, unlike most other glutamate receptor-channels, is permeable to calcium ions. Inappropriate activation of this receptor induces toxic levels of intracellular calcium which can ultimately lead to cell death (this toxic mechanism, termed excitotoxicity, is largely responsible for the brain damage induced by ischaemia and stroke). On the island of Guam in the Indian Ocean, there is a high incidence of a neurological disorder, called Guam disease, which resembles many of the features of Parkinson's disease, Alzheimer's disease and motor neuron disease – all brain disorders associated with the death of neurons. It appears that the most likely cause of Guam disease is the use of the cycad nut in the local cuisine – a nut which contains a powerful agonist at the NMDA receptor. You will learn more about the physiological and cognitive processes that utilize NMDA receptors in Book 5, Chapter 1; particularly those processes involved in modifying neural networks.

Neuropeptides

Neuro-active peptides (**neuropeptides**) are involved in the signalling of mood and pain. In some neurons, they are synthesized in the presynaptic cells (and serve as a neurotransmitter). However, they are often synthesized elsewhere, even outside the brain in glands such as the pancreas, or in the heart and gut. They enter the brain in the bloodstream and then diffuse into groups of neurons. Acting in this way they can affect large numbers of neurons simultaneously. Such an effect is therefore rather different from that of a neurotransmitter where activity is restricted to the synapse. Rather, the role of neuropeptides is to cause changes in the sensitivity of reactivity of whole populations of neurons to neurotransmission. For this reason peptides function as neuromodulators (see Section 1.6.3). Studies of neuromodulators have greatly increased our understanding of brain function. They can alter the transmission of signals across synapses in a variety of ways, by increasing or decreasing the release of neurotransmitter, or by changing the properties of postsynaptic receptors. It is now known that many neurons synthesize peptide transmitters in addition to one or other of the 'classic' neurotransmitters described above.

Neuropeptides, such as substance P, the enkephalins and the endorphins are believed to be neurotransmitters in the accepted sense in that they are synthesized and released by cells at synapses.

Enkephalins and endorphins belong to a class of peptide neurotransmitter called endogenous opioids. The term 'endogenous' refers to the fact that they are made naturally within the body. Opioids act on opiate receptors, which can also be stimulated by both legal and illegal means. Narcotic opiate drugs produce their analgesic and euphoria-inducing effects by acting at these same receptor sites. The analgesia refers to a capacity to reduce the sensation of pain. Morphine is one of the better known examples of a drug in this class and is prescribed to reduce severe pain.

Cannabinoids

Cannabis is a substance that is widely used by individuals to promote feelings of euphoria and exhilaration, though it can also impair short-term memory and induce paranoia. It is believed to have originated in central Asia, probably in China. The earliest historical reference to cannabis dates back over 4000 years to a legendary Chinese emperor named Chen Nung. Western interest in cannabis did not begin until the early middle 19th century, when some of Napoleon's soldiers brought it back to France from Egypt.

Cannabis is derived from the flowering hemp plant and comes in several forms including marijuana and hashish. The active compound in cannabis has been indentified as tetrahydrocannabinol (THC). Whilst THC is not itself a neurotransmitter, the use of radiolabelled THC has revealed the presence of cannabinoid receptors in the brain; particularly in the hippocampus, a brain region involved in short-term memory (see Book 1, Section 3.4.4 and Book 5, Chapter 1). The discovery of these cannabinoid receptors initiated the search for the endogenous agonist – the body's own form of 'cannabis'. Since 1992, several compounds have been identified as endogenous agonists at cannabinoid receptors, all derived from the fatty acid, arachidonate. The first compound isolated was arachidonylethanolamide and has been named 'anandamide', from *ananda*, the Sanskrit word for 'bliss'.

Despite the whimsical name given to this naturally occurring compound, very little is known about how these endogenous agonists are regulated, though their receptors may provide a new route to treating several brain disorders, including Alzheimer's disease, and alleviating the pain associated with multiple sclerosis.

1.5   Neuronal integration

1.5.1   The neuron as an information processor

The output of a neuron is the action potential. The function of the synaptic input onto any given neuron is to 'determine' if that neuron will generate an action potential or, if it is already spontaneously active, to modify the pattern and frequency of action potential firing. Before we discuss how a neuron integrates synaptic activity to produce an output, we should first consider how excitatory and inhibitory synaptic potentials (EPSPs and IPSPs) differ from the action potential. Unlike action potentials, EPSPs and IPSPs are not all-or-nothing events. If you recall from Section 1.3.1, once a cell is depolarized sufficiently to reach the firing threshold (usually at the axon hillock), the action potential ensues and is propagated throughout the cell by the recruitment of voltage-dependent sodium channels. An EPSP or IPSP is generated by the opening of neurotransmitter-gated ion channels located at the synapses on the postsynaptic membrane. The current generated by these transiently open channels spreads along the membrane but, unlike an action potential which is propagated by a wave of channel opening, the voltage change gradually decays back to the resting membrane potential (see Figure 1.17). A single excitatory synapse is unlikely to generate sufficient depolarization to bring a cell to its firing threshold. In order to evoke an action potential, several excitatory synaptic inputs must act together. In terms of processing information, this represents the addition or 'summation' of the inputs to the neuron. Whether or not an action potential arises in the postsynaptic cell depends on the total amount of depolarization.

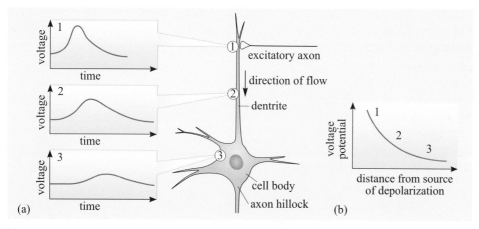

Figure 1.17   (a) Schematic showing a cell with a single dendrite (for simplicity) with an excitatory input. EPSP traces corresponding to points 1, 2 and 3 marked on the cell show how the EPSP decays as it travels from the distal dendrite to the cell body. (b) A graph showing the decay of a synaptic potential.

Temporal summation is the term used to describe the integration of incoming signals to the postsynaptic cell with respect to time. Figure 1.18 shows an example of this. Activation of an excitatory synapse by an action potential causes an EPSP. If another action potential arrives sufficiently soon after the first, there will be an addition of the EPSPs with the result that the magnitude of the depolarization is greater than that produced by a single action potential alone.

Figure 1.18   Temporal summation of synaptic input. (a) If the time interval between the two action potentials is sufficiently large (t_1) two distinct EPSPs are seen. (b) If the action potentials are closer together in time (t_2), the EPSP produced by the first has not decayed to zero at the time the second occurs – summation results.

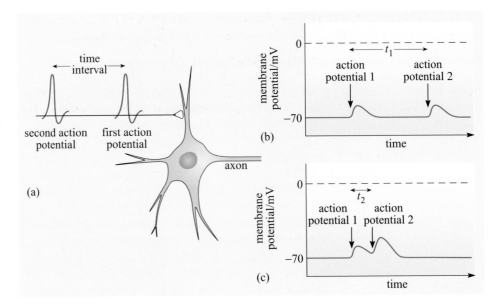

◆   What determines if two EPSPs, generated by the same presynaptic terminal, will undergo temporal summation?

◆   In order for two EPSPs to summate, they must overlap – the arrival of the two action potentials at the presynaptic terminal must be close enough together in time to ensure that the EPSP generated by the first is still present when the second action potential initiates the second EPSP.

Spatial summation is the process whereby a neuron integrates the effects of synapses at different locations on the cell. The principle is the same as for temporal summation and is illustrated in Figure 1.19.

Figure 1.19   Spatial summation of synaptic input. (a) A neuron (cell 3) with two excitatory synapses made with presynaptic neurons 1 and 2. (b) The effect at the axon hillock of neuron 3 of the synaptic potential produced by activation of neuron 1, the synaptic potential produced by activation of neuron 2 and the synaptic potential produced by simultaneous activation of neurons 1 and 2 – resulting in spatial summation.

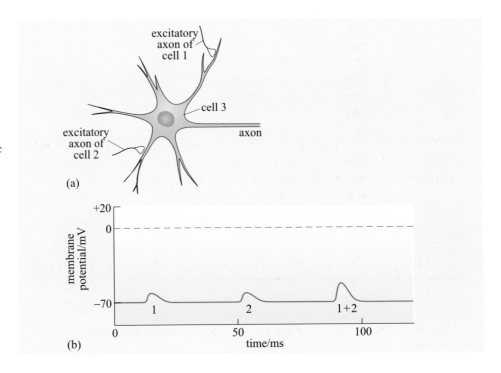

◆ Look at Figure 1.19. What is the effect at the axon hillock of the postsynaptic cell of action potentials arriving from both neurons 1 and 2 simultaneously?

◆ An additive effect on the size of the EPSP.

Figure 1.20 shows a neuron with both excitatory and inhibitory synapses, and the effect of action potentials arriving at each input both separately and simultaneously.

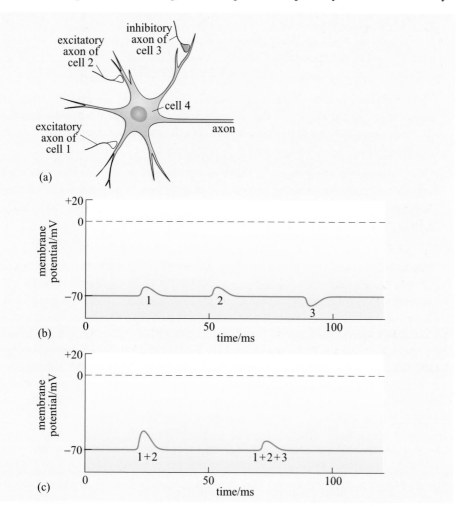

(a)

(b)

(c)

Figure 1.20 Synaptic integration. (a) Two excitatory (1 and 2) and one inhibitory (3) synapses are made upon a neuron (cell 4). (b) The change in membrane potential caused by stimulating each presynaptic neuron in turn. (c) The effect of stimulating 1 and 2 simultaneously and then 1, 2 and 3 simultaneously.

◆ What is the effect in cell 4 of the simultaneous arrival of action potentials from neurons 1 and 2?

◆ An EPSP that is greater than those of either 1 or 2 individually.

◆ What is the effect in cell 4 of action potentials arriving simultaneously at the excitatory synapses 1 and 2 and the inhibitory synapse 3?

◆ An EPSP is generated, but it is smaller than the EPSP that would be produced by the summation of 1 and 2. Activity in synapse 3 acts in the opposite direction to activity in 1 and 2.

A neuron might have many excitatory and inhibitory synapses activated simultaneously.

◆   What determines the magnitude of the change in polarization in the postsynaptic cell?

◆   It is determined by the balance of activity in excitatory and inhibitory presynaptic neurons. The number of inputs is important: depolarization is more likely the larger the number of active excitatory inputs and the fewer the number of inhibitory inputs. Also the distance from the axon hillock will affect the effectiveness of each input (look again at Figure 1.17b).

So far, in terms of synaptic integration, we have assumed that synaptic activity is targeted to the postsynaptic cell. The control of the release of transmitter from an axon terminal is also an important step for regulating the flow of information.

1   Some inhibitory neurons make synaptic connections directly on the presynaptic terminal or on the axon near the terminal – these synapses when activated can prevent the release of neurotransmitter from the presynaptic terminal. (See the example of an axo-axonic synapse shown in Figure 1.12.)

2   Some presynaptic terminals also have receptors that are activated by the release of neurotransmitter from the terminal – such receptors are called autoreceptors. Some autoreceptors terminate transmitter release, others augment it.

1.5.2   The neural code and neurotransmitter release

As mentioned earlier, the action potential represents the output signal of the neuron. The frequency and pattern of action potential firing will have a profound effect on the amount of neurotransmitter released at the axon terminals. An example of this is illustrated in Figure 1.21. The neuron shown in Figure 1.21 is a sensory neuron; a cell that has a specialized ending (receptor site) that is sensitive to stretch (such cells respond to touch). Deformation of this sensory ending, by stretching, opens stretch-sensitive ion channels that depolarize the neuron, in much the same way that an excitatory neurotransmitter released from a presynaptic terminal elicits an EPSP. To distinguish this type of excitatory potential from an EPSP, it is called a **receptor potential**.

◆   Look at Figure 1.21. What determines the size of the receptor potential?

◆   The amplitude and duration of the receptor potential is determined by the amplitude and duration of the sensory stimulus, in this case the stretch.

The depolarizing receptor potential spreads down the sensory neuron until it reaches a specialized portion of the membrane called the trigger zone; its function is very much like that of the axon hillock discussed earlier. At the trigger zone the receptor potential is converted into action potentials, the number and frequency of action potentials is directly related to the amplitude and duration of the receptor potential – and the amount of neurotransmitter released at the axon terminals of the sensory neuron is a function of the number and frequency of action potentials generated.

Some neurons such as those that release the neurotransmitters dopamine or serotonin (neurotransmitters that affect mood, arousal and our sense of well-being)

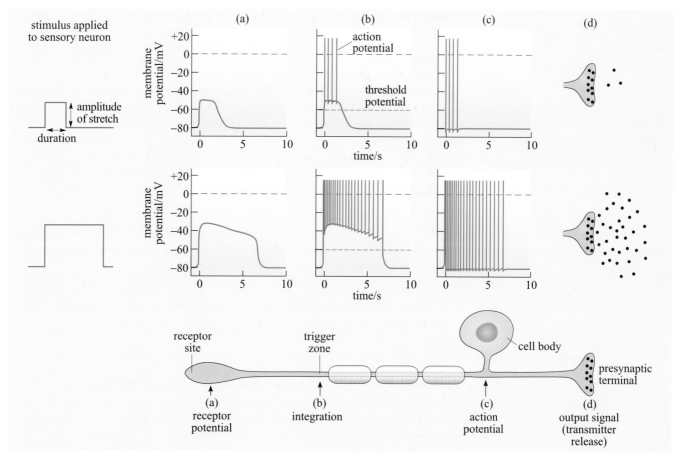

Figure 1.21 Relationship between firing rate and release of neurotransmitter. A sensory neuron transforms sensory stimuli (in this example stretches of different amplitudes and durations) into electrical activity in the cell. (a) The input signal is graded in amplitude and duration, proportional to the amplitude and duration of the stimulus. (b) The trigger zone transforms the input signal into action potentials that will be propagated along the axon. An action potential is generated only if the receptor potential (or in the case of a synapse, the EPSP) is greater than the threshold potential. Once the input signal surpasses the threshold potential, any further increase in amplitude of the input signal increases the frequency with which the action potentials are generated. Thus the graded nature of the input signals is translated into a frequency code of action potentials. (c) The action potentials are propagated along the axon. (d) When the action potential reaches the synaptic terminal, the neurotransmitter is released. The total number of action potentials per unit time (frequency) determines the amount of neurotransmitter released – more action potentials mean a greater amount of neurotransmitter will be released.

fire action potentials spontaneously and continuously (1 to 20 times per second), producing a steady stream (*tonic release*) of neurotransmitter. Other neurons, such as the glutamatergic (glutamate releasing) pyramidal neurons of the cerebral cortex (involved in the control of movement, abstract thought and the processing of complex information), require the action of excitatory synaptic inputs in order to bring them to their firing threshold. Often neurons produce bursts of action potentials in response to a stimulus, releasing large quantities of neurotransmitter in a very short time. The frequency of action potential firing can be modified by neurotransmitters. Figure 1.22 demonstrates the powerful excitatory effect of the neurotransmitter, noradrenalin, on the firing properties of a cortical neuron and the effect that an IPSP has on the firing rate of a tonically active dopaminergic neuron located in the substantia nigra.

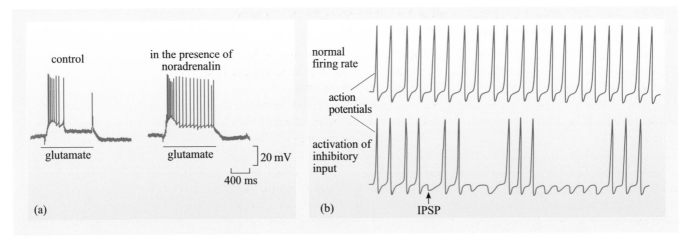

Figure 1.22   (a) The effect of exogenous application of the neurotransmitter, noradrenalin, on the firing rate of a hippocampal pyramidal neuron recorded using an intracellular electrode. The cell is depolarized to its firing threshold by the application of the neurotransmitter glutamate which excites the cell by activating excitatory glutamate receptors located on the cell. (b) The upper trace shows the spontaneous generation of action potentials in a dopaminergic neuron. The lower trace shows the inhibitory effect of a single IPSP on the pattern of action potential generation.

Excitatory neurotransmitters are not the only means of evoking action potentials. Our bodies contain a host of sensory receptors that convey information about the outside world (e.g. photoreceptors in the eye used for vision) and the internal world (e.g. osmoreceptors – receptors that are sensitive to changes in water concentration in the brain that regulate thirst). These receptors, in response to sensory or physical stimuli, can either generate action potentials themselves (where the receptor is a specialized neuron like the stretch sensitive neuron shown in Figure 1.21) or release signalling molecules that induce synaptic responses in nearby neurons: receptors are said to act as *transducers* – turning physical stimuli into an electrical response. We have already met an example of sensory transduction in the form of the stretch sensitive sensory neuron illustrated in Figure 1.21. Here, a physical stimulus (stretch) is transformed into an electrical response.

Synaptic summation is an integrative property of the postsynaptic membrane. The presynaptic terminal is also capable of integrative processing. If you recall from Section 1.4.3, neurotransmitter release is triggered by the entry of calcium ions into the presynaptic terminal in response to the depolarization produced by the invading action potential. Whilst the rise in calcium concentration is transient, it still requires several milliseconds for the calcium concentration to return to its former level. If a second action potential should invade the presynaptic terminal during this period, the calcium that enters the terminal is added to the residual calcium still present in the terminal and more neurotransmitter is released (i.e. neurotransmitter release is proportional to the amount of calcium present in the axon terminal).

Summary of Sections 1.4 and 1.5

Messages are passed across synapses by chemical transmitter molecules called neurotransmitters (except in the case of electrical synapses, where gap junctions allow the direct passage of ions from cell to cell). The arrival of an action potential at the presynaptic terminal causes the intracellular calcium concentration to increase locally, and this in turn triggers the release of neurotransmitter molecules from the

synaptic vesicles. Reuptake mechanisms allow neurotransmitter molecules to be recaptured and thereby released and reused many times over.

The postsynaptic membrane contains receptor molecules that, by virtue of their shape, are specific for a particular neurotransmitter with a complementary shape (the lock and key). Binding of neurotransmitter to a postsynaptic receptor opens ion channels in the postsynaptic membrane. Some receptor molecules are themselves ion channels (direct) but others stimulate the production of second messengers with the postsynaptic cell – these second messengers may lead to the opening or closure of ion channels (indirect) or mediate other events in the cell. Receptors can be distinguished by their binding of pharmacological agonists and antagonists. Agonists mimic the effect of the natural neurotransmitter whereas antagonists inhibit the functioning of the receptor. Neurotransmitter binding to an excitatory receptor produces an EPSP whereas neurotransmitter binding to an inhibitory receptor produces an IPSP. Temporal and spatial summation are the mechanisms by which the postsynaptic cell integrates all the various incoming signals.

1.6 Wiring the brain

1.6.1 Building a neural processor

So far we have considered how the output of a neuron is influenced by the balance of activity in inhibitory and excitatory inputs on that cell. Now we will consider how neurons operate together to convey information.

The simplest information processor is a system that converts a physical stimulus into a behavioural response – such an example is seen in the stretch response (Book 1, Section 3.3.2) and is illustrated in Figure 1.23. Here a stretch-sensitive neuron (this neuron has a special stretch receptor which is part of a *muscle spindle* – you will learn more about these in Chapter 2 of this book) is synaptically connected to a second neuron (a motor neuron) capable of exciting a muscle. In this simple reflex circuit, stimulation of the sensory neuron generates an action potential in the sensory neuron that leads to excitation of the motor neuron, which in turn causes the muscle to twitch.

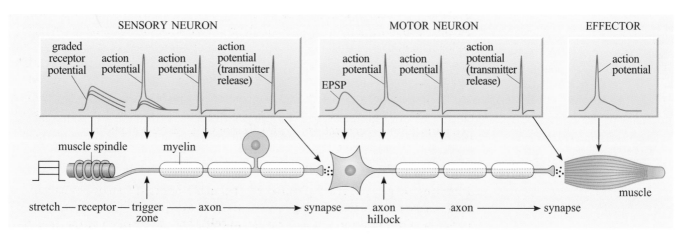

Figure 1.23 A stretch-sensitive neuron (the afferent neuron) makes a direct excitatory connection to a motor neuron (the efferent neuron). The upper traces show the potentials recorded along the length of the circuit.

◆ The same result could be achieved by simply connecting the sensory neuron directly to the muscle. What advantage does the synapse give?

◆ The addition of a synapse to the circuit introduces a site for modifying the reflex response.

A sensory reflex is rarely as simple as that shown in Figure 1.23. The reflex circuitry is part of larger neural network with both local and higher control systems (see the description of spinal reflexes in in Book 1, Section 3.3.2). Continuous activation of the sensory neuron in Figure 1.23 will produce a maintained excitation of the muscle via the motor neuron – a situation that if allowed to persist, could result in damage to the muscle.

◆ How would you modify the simple circuit discussed above to prevent damage to the muscle?

◆ One solution is to introduce an inhibitory interneuron to reduce activity in the motor neuron.

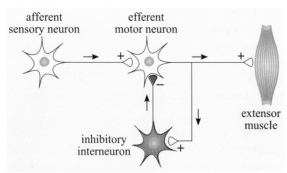

Figure 1.24   A sensory neuron makes an excitatory connection with a motor neuron (similar to that shown in Figure 1.23). However, unlike the circuit shown in Figure 1.23, the motor neuron also makes an excitatory connection with an inhibitory interneuron. In turn, the inhibitory interneuron feeds back onto the motor neuron by making an inhibitory synaptic connection with it – so activation of the motor neuron will also activate an inhibitory feedback loop via the inhibitory interneuron, limiting both the excitatory effect of the sensory input and the output of the motor neuron. This form of negative feedback is therefore self-regulating.

Figure 1.24 shows a neural circuit similar to the one discussed above but in addition it also contains an inhibitory interneuron. The motor neuron, as well as being connected to the muscle, also makes an excitatory synaptic connection (indicated by a +) to an inhibitory interneuron which in turn makes an inhibitory connection with the motor neuron (indicated by a −). So, under these conditions, activity in the motor neuron results in an increase in the inhibitory input, thereby reducing the ability of the circuit to cause sustained and potentially damaging contraction of the muscle. This is an example of **feedback inhibition** and demonstrates how the addition of an extra neuronal component to a network can radically alter the properties of that network. (The term *feedback* is used because the inhibitory input inhibits the neural circuit that activated the inhibitory interneuron; in other words, the inhibitory input feeds back onto its excitatory source. In the case of the circuit shown in Figure 1.24, the excitatory source is the motor neuron.) As well as limiting activity within its own immediate circuit, inhibitory interneurons can influence activity in adjacent, and often competing, neural circuits; a phenonomen called **feedforward inhibition**. Figure 1.25 illustrates an example of feedforward inhibition used to regulate the activation of flexor and extensor muscles. (These are muscle groups that work in opposition to each other – the extensor muscles of the arm, for example, extend the arm whilst the flexor muscles flex it. If both groups of muscles were activated at the same time, the result would be a rigid arm – an arm that could not move!) Here, the sensory or afferent input activates an inhibitory neuron that inhibits activity in a parallel neural circuit but not its own circuit – you were introduced to reciprocal innervation in Book 1, Chapter 3 (also see Figure 3.8 in Book 1).

Our understanding of the complex array of neural networks that make up a human brain is still at a rudimentary level. However, some insight has been gained from the study of patients that have suffered forms of brain injury or insult. Such injuries often induce abnormal forms of behaviour and disturbed mental function. For

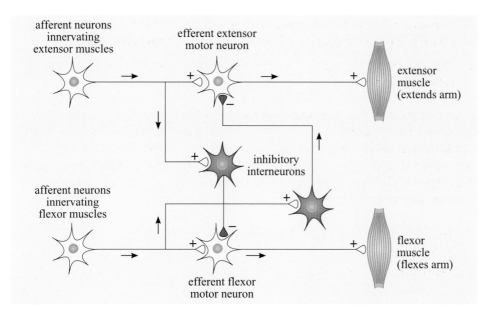

afferent neurons
innervating
extensor muscles

efferent extensor
motor neuron

extensor
muscle
(extends arm)

inhibitory
interneurons

afferent neurons
innervating
flexor muscles

flexor
muscle
(flexes arm)

efferent flexor
motor neuron

Figure 1.25 Afferent neurons from extensor muscles excite not only the extensor motor neurons, but also inhibitory interneurons that prevent the firing of the motor neurons in the opposing flexor muscles. Feedforward inhibition enhances the effect of the active pathways by suppressing the activity of the other, opposing pathways.

example, the paralysis often associated with stroke patients is caused by damage to the motor cortex. Stroke-induced lesions (areas of cell loss; see Book 1, Box 3.4) alter the flow of information within the motor neural networks, producing aberrant outcomes such as poor coordination of movement or paralysis. As you will learn later, the selective loss of particular subsets of neurons can have widespread implications for brain function. For the moment, imagine what would happen even in a simple circuit such as those illustrated in Figures 1.24 and 1.25 should the inhibitory interneurons die or become dysfunctional.

Before we broaden our discussion to consider the role of more complex neural circuits, it is important to appreciate that not all neural function or behaviour is regulated by sensory input. Our brains have entire neural networks dedicated to processing abstract thought, processes which are not necessarily dependent on the physical and sensory world – though of course, these networks are very much connected to them, and can and do interact with these other systems.

1.6.2 Cerebellum and cerebral cortex: neural processors

You should now have an appreciation of how relatively simple components, such as excitatory and inhibitory neurons and their synaptic connections, can be combined to produce very complex and elaborate networks (also look again at the examples mentioned in Book 1, in Chapters 2 and 3). At one level, we can view these networks as being hard-wired circuits, very much like the circuits found in a computer. Neural networks have evolved that process particular forms of information and they often possess distinct neuronal cell types with specific integrative properties. Figure 1.26 illustrates some of the neural networks found in human brains. Each performs a very different role, has different patterns of innervation and possesses their own unique neuronal forms. (You will learn more about the function of these brain regions as you progress through the course.) The common denominator for each network is that they all use synaptic integration to modify action potential generation resulting in an interplay of chemical and electrical signalling.

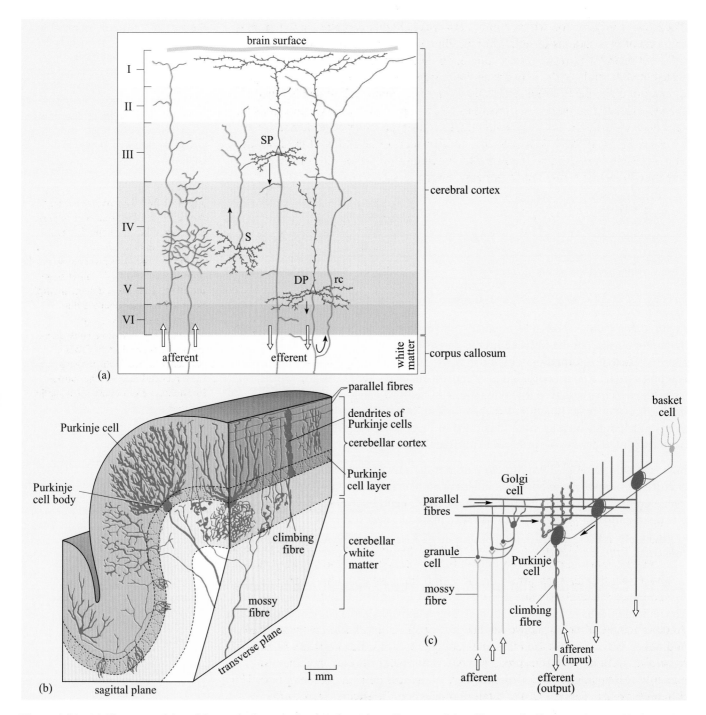

Figure 1.26 (a) The connectivity of the cerebral cortex showing the major cell types and the efferent and afferent pathways. The layered distribution of cell types (the cell bodies are shown) through the six layers of the cortex. (S = stellate cell, SP = superficial pyramidal cell, DP = deep pyramid cell, rc = recurrent collateral axon.) Dendrites are shown in red and axons in brown. (b) The distribution and cell types found in the cerebellum. (c) The major afferent input onto the Purkinje cells is from the parallel fibres and climbing fibres. Note how the parallel fibre input converges onto the Purkinje cells, the output neurons of the cerebellum.

The flow of information within neural networks is highly complex, but often falls into one of two patterns of organization. Figure 1.27 shows examples of these different neural templates. Information entering a network can be dispersed; distributed throughout the network so that a single neuron can influence a large number of cells; the information is said to *diverge* (Figure 1.27a) and is often a feature of neural networks that process sensory input. Conversely, many cells may terminate on a single neuron (Figure 1.27b). This type of network demonstrates the *convergence* of neural information and is often seen at the output of the nervous system. By receiving signals from multiple neurons, the target cell is able to integrate diverse information from many sources.

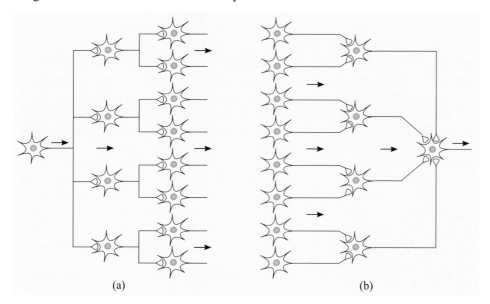

(a)   (b)

Figure 1.27 The divergence and convergence of neuronal connections represent a key principle in the organization of the brain.
(a) Divergence. In sensory systems the receptor neurons at the input stage usually branch out and make multiple connections with neurons that represent the second stage of information processing, subsequent connections can diverge further.
(b) Convergence. With convergence, the target cell receives the sum of information from many presynaptic neurons.

◆ Look at Figure 1.26c, what type of network best describes the pattern of input onto the Purkinje cells of the cerebellum?

◆ The Purkinje cells represent the major output cell of the cerebellum. These cells receive a convergent input from both the parallel fibres and to a lesser extent, also from the climbing fibres. Purkinje cells integrate the output from a *convergent* neural network.

Another feature of neural networks that greatly enhances their processing speed and power is that information is processed by many neurons or groups of neurons in parallel, i.e. many neurons process similar information at the same time. An example of a neural network that uses parallel processing is the visual system. Here, different groups of cells are dedicated to processing different aspects of the sensory input; each processing a particular element, such as movement, distance, colour, contrast, luminosity, orientation, direction of movement, etc. This information is then seamlessly combined to give a visual image. Without parallel processing, our visual experience would be very limited.

1.6.3 Networks and neurotransmitters

Another way to look at neural networks is not to think of them as physical structures simply involved in the initiation and conduction of action potentials, but instead, to think of them as a system of competing and complementary

neurotransmitter networks (this will be explained further in the next section). The major excitatory and inhibitory neurotransmitters in the brain are the amino acids glutamate and GABA respectively. These neurotransmitters evoke rapid synaptic potentials by acting primarily on directly gated ion channels and they also mediate activity within neural networks. (This is of course an oversimplification as the action of glutamate and GABA is not restricted to directly gated ion channels. These neurotransmitters also activate indirectly gated ion channels.) Overlying this largely amino acid-based neurotransmitter network are other neurotransmitter systems, namely the dopaminergic, serotonergic and noradrenergic networks that have powerful **neuromodulatory** effects (Box 1.1), such as increasing the excitability of a cell so that the likelihood of an excitatory input eliciting an action potential is increased, or modulating the release of neurotransmitter from the presynaptic terminal. Axon terminals releasing these modulatory neurotransmitters often arise from discrete populations of neurons located in distinct nuclei as illustrated in Figure 1.28. These cells send axons throughout the brain, innervating multiple brain structures and, depending on the types of receptors present at the postsynaptic targets, these axons can exert both inhibitory and excitatory responses (Box 1.2). A structural feature of these neuromodulatory systems is that instead of releasing their neurotransmitter from discrete axon terminals, such as the presynaptic terminal shown in Figure 1.13, they often employ a less 'precise' structure called a varicosity. A varicosity is a swelling in the axon that contains synaptic vesicles (an axon can have many varicosities along its length) that upon activation, by an action potential passing along the axon, release their neurotransmitter into the local vicinity. The utility of a varicosity is that once released, the neurotransmitter is not restricted to the presynaptic cleft, but diffuses into the surrounding tissue where it has the potential to influence many cells.

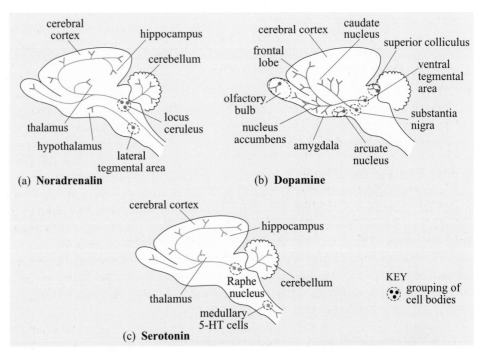

Figure 1.28   The projection pathways and nuclei are shown for the (a) noradrenergic, (b) dopaminergic and (c) serotonergic neurotransmitter systems (in this case, for the rat brain). Note how they arise from discrete populations of cells (nuclei; indicated by dotted circles) and that the projection pathways differ for each neurotransmitter system. (5-HT is serotonin.)

Box 1.2   More neurotransmitters

Amines

Acetylcholine (ACh) was the first neurotransmitter to be discovered by Dale in 1914. Cholinergic neurons (neurons which release ACh as their neurotransmitter) are particularly abundant in the basal ganglia, and others seem to be involved in cortical arousal. The loss of cholinergic neurons is one of the major causes of Alzheimer's disease. Acetylcholine is mainly an excitatory neurotransmitter. It is released by motor neurons at the neuromuscular junction (the synapse made between a motor neuron and muscle) where it acts on nicotinic receptors (named for their sensitivity for the tobacco plant extract, nicotine) to excite muscle. The excitatory effects of ACh in the central nervous system are usually mediated via another type of ACh receptor, the muscarinic receptors (named for their sensitivity to the mushroom extract, muscarine).

Acetylcholine is rapidly removed from the synaptic cleft or neuromuscular junction by the degradative action of an enzyme called acetycholinesterase (AChE).

Catecholamines is the generic name for the family of neurotransmitters containing both **dopamine** and **noradrenalin** – often referred to (together with serotonin and adrenalin) as the biogenic amines. These neurotransmitters have a similar chemical structure and share a common synthesizing pathway. They are synthesized from the amino acids tyrosine and phenylalanine. Tyrosine enters the catecholaminergic neuron directly from the bloodstream, or it can be made from phenylalanine by enzymes within the cell. Inside the cell, tyrosine is converted into l-dopa and then into dopamine. You will read in Section 1.6.4 how levodopa, a precursor for dopamine, is used to raise levels of dopamine in the treatment of Parkinson's disease. Noradrenergic neurons convert dopamine into noradrenalin (neurons that release adrenalin go one step further and convert noradrenalin into adrenalin).

Dopamine occurs in pathways essential for sensory and motor performance. It induces euphoria and has also been implicated in drug addiction, particularly drugs of abuse such as cocaine which facilitates the release of dopamine from dopaminergic terminals. Only a small percentage of the neurons in the brain synthesize dopamine, yet these neurons by means of their extensive network of axon terminals, can influence function in most brain regions. In Section

1.6.4 you will learn that a deficiency of dopamine in the basal ganglia leads to the loss of motor control.

Noradrenalin is one of the most important neurotransmitters in determining the capacity of the body to exhibit 'fight or flight' behaviour in the face of danger. It has both excitatory and inhibitory effects in the central nervous system. In the brain, noradrenalin is synthesized by a few highly branched neurons (see Figure 1.28) and is involved in many aspects of brain function. Overstimulation of the noradrenergic system leads to symptoms of mania and the neurotransmitter is also known to be involved in feeding and drinking.

Adrenalin is synthetized by neurons in the brain and by a gland called the adrenal gland (see Book 1, Section 3.5.1). When secreted into the bloodstream it acts as a circulating hormone often known as the 'fight or flight' hormone (Book 1, Box 3.3). However, as a neurotransmitter in the nervous system, it can have *either* excitatory or inhibitory effects. It is involved in the regulation of body temperature, blood pressure and respiratory rate.

Serotonin (5-hydroxytryptamine, 5-HT) occurs in neuronal cell bodies of the Raphe nucleus of the brainstem which project to many forebrain areas and spinal cord (See Figure 1.28). Serotonin is implicated in the sleep/wake cycle, temperature regulation, control of aggressive behaviour, sexual activity and modulation of pain. Serotonin may, together with noradrenalin, be involved in depression. Drugs which prevent the reuptake of serotonin, such as 'Ecstasy' (MDMA; 3,4-methylenedioxymethamphetamine) are widely used as recreational mood enhancers. Users say that Ecstasy lowers their inhibitions and relaxes them. It is also reported to heighten awareness and feelings of pleasure and to give people energy. Other effects include headaches, chills, eye twitching, jaw clenching, blurred vision and nausea. In extreme cases, Ecstasy can cause dehydration, hyperthermia, seizures and death. As this course goes to press, the growing recreational use of Ecstasy is the subject of much debate. There is growing and disturbing evidence that the use of Ecstasy can lead to long-term damage to the serotonergic and dopaminergic neural networks; possibly leading to the development in later life of psychiatric illnesses such as depression, schizophrenia and possibly, Parkinson's disease.

1.6.4 The basal ganglia: a neural network at work

Understanding how neural networks process information, respond and communicate with other brain systems is one of the current research goals in neuroscience. At first glance, a neural circuit can look daunting. One approach to unravelling this complexity is to think about how the output of the network (behaviour) is affected by alterations in the balance of activity in the different neurotransmitter systems involved. An example of how one can use this approach to understand network function is in the basal ganglia.

The basal ganglia are made up of a number of subcortical structures that include the striatum (containing the putamen and caudate nucleus), the internal and external segments of the globus pallidus, the subthalamic nucleus and the substantia nigra (see Book 1, Figure 3.11). Figure 1.29 is a schematic diagram showing the major wiring pathways of the basal ganglia – the connections between these structures are very complex and have been greatly simplified to aid understanding. The functions of the basal ganglia are not fully understood but there is growing evidence that they are involved in the control of movement; particularly planning and motor strategy. Most of the information we have about their function comes from clinical observations of human patients with subcortical lesions (areas of cell loss); the best known examples come from Parkinson's disease and Huntington's disease (mentioned in Book 1, Sections 1.5.2 and 3.4.4).

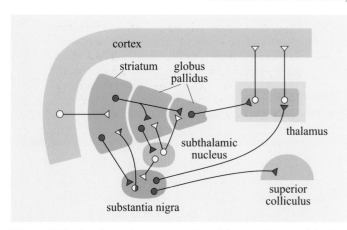

Figure 1.29   A schematic representation of the neural network in the basal ganglia. The basal ganglia is a collection of interconnected populations of neurons that are involved in the control and planning of motor activity. The figure shows some of these neuronal groupings and the connections made by them. Inhibitory cell bodies and synapses are represented in red; excitatory cell bodies are white. Endings that are both white and red indicate that the neurotransmitter released can have either an excitatory or inhibitory action on the presynaptic neuron.

Parkinson's disease is due to the selective loss of the output dopaminergic neurons of the substantia nigra. The causes of Parkinson's disease are not fully understood but the effect it has on patients is devastating, gradually robbing them of their ability to control or initiate movement. The main feature of classic Parkinson's disease is a general loss of movement (akinesia). Patients lose the ability to make normal facial expressions, consequently they appear lifeless and apathetic. They may blink less often than a normal individual; there is often a shuffling gait, and they may be very slow in walking. None of the above is a defect of the peripheral motor system or muscles, for under the right circumstances, especially under strong emotional stimulation, quite normal movements can be made. For example, a person with Parkinson's disease may be shuffling his way across a road when a car comes along. He then runs briskly to the other side of the road to avoid an accident, but as soon as he reaches the safety of the pavement, he resumes his shuffling gait. The difficulty, in other words, is not in the execution of the movement but in its initiation. Other common features of Parkinson's disease are a general rigidity and slowness (bradykinesia), inappropriate posture and tremor (known as a *rest* tremor), all associated with altered neural processing within the basal ganglia. Also, patients may exhibit cognitive and emotional disorders. Parkinson's disease can be said to be a hypokinetic condition (too little activity).

On the other hand, Huntington's disease is a hyperkinetic disorder (too much motor activity). Patients exhibit poorly controlled exaggerated movements, pronounced tremor and erratic dance-like movements (chorea). Huntington's disease is due, in part, to the loss of GABAergic neurons of the striatum.

If we now look at the basal ganglia, not so much in terms of the afferent and efferent connections made between different subcortical structures, but as a series of neurotransmitter systems, it then becomes possible to make some working assumptions about information flow between their different structures. The three key neurotransmitters, in terms of balance of activity within the basal ganglia, appear to be dopamine, acetylcholine (ACh) and GABA.

Figure 1.30 shows how these neurotransmitter systems are believed to interact to regulate the outflow of information into the motor network (thalamus, cortex and spinal cord). The dopaminergic neurons of the substantia nigra, which are tonically active (Figure 1.22b shows an example of a tonically active dopaminergic neuron), project to the striatum where they make inhibitory synaptic connections onto a subpopulation of cholinergic neurons. These neurons then make excitatory connections onto the output GABAergic neurons of the striatum, which in turn send a projection back to the substantia nigra to inhibit the dopaminergic system. In a normal individual, it is believed that the dopaminergic and GABAergic systems are in some form of functional equilibrium. However, in Parkinson's disease and Huntington's disease this equilibrium is disturbed and results in abnormal output from the basal ganglia and consequently motor behaviour is also abnormal. The loss of dopamine in Parkinson's disease increases the GABAergic output of the striatum whereas a decrease in GABA, commonly seen in Huntington's disease, increases the release of dopamine from the substantia nigra.

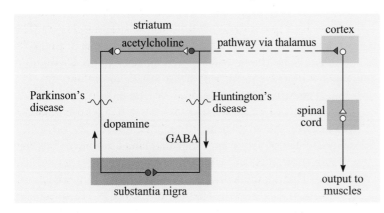

Figure 1.30 Schematic representation of the balance of activity between the neurotransmitters dopamine, acetylcholine and GABA. Parkinson's disease affects the dopamine pathway whilst Huntington's disease affects the GABA output of the striatum. Inhibitory cell bodies and synapses are represented in red; excitatory cell bodies and synapses are white.

◆ Can you describe hypokinesia and hyperkinesia in terms of dopamine levels in the basal ganglia?

◆ Hypokinesia is due to too little dopamine whereas hyperkinesia is due to too much dopamine.

The treatment of these conditions, using drugs, has focused on trying to restore the normal level of dopaminergic activity in the basal ganglia.

◆ How might a drug be used to restore the normal levels of dopamine in Parkinson's disease?

◆ Drugs could be used to increase dopamine levels by (i) increasing its synthesis, (ii) increasing its release from dopaminergic cells, (iii) inhibiting its removal from the extracellular fluid. All of the above can be achieved by using drugs given to the patient orally or by injection – however, dopamine itself is of limited use as it does not readily pass through the blood–brain barrier (see Book 1, Section 3.5.2) and it is also rapidly inactivated in the body.

In combating Parkinson's disease, medical practice is targeted to raising the levels of dopamine. One approach is to enhance the synthesis of dopamine in the surviving dopaminergic neurons by giving the patients large doses of the dopamine precursor molecule, levodopa (l-dopa). Precursor molecules are molecules that are used in the synthesis of other molecules. Levodopa is used because it can be administered orally (taken by mouth) and importantly, it can cross the blood–brain barrier. Drugs that inhibit the reuptake of dopamine, prevents its inactivation or facilitate its release from the terminal can also be helpful in raising the extracellular levels of dopamine. Alternatively, drugs that block the action of acetylcholine released from the striatal cholinergic neurons have shown some efficacy in the treatment of Parkinson's disease. However, none of these pharmacological interventions prevent the progression of the underlying disease, they only, for a time, restore the balance of activity within the basal ganglia.

Another approach to treating Parkinson's disease is to regulate the output from the basal ganglia by using stimulating electrodes to impose an ordered pattern of neuronal firing that resembles the pattern seen in normal subjects (a therapy called deep brain stimulation (DBS), first mentioned in Book 3, Section 2.4.1). The elegance of this approach is that the rate and intensity of stimulation is finely tuned to the patient – in some cases, deep brain stimulation can bring about instantaneous relief of the motor components of the disease.

◆ What advantage does deep brain stimulation have over drug therapies in the treatment of Parkinson's disease?

◆ A problem with most drug therapies is specificity of action, in terms of brain region and unwanted interactions at other sites of action. Deep brain stimulation restores motor function by targeting the output of the basal ganglia, and this is achieved in an anatomical and therefore a highly specific manner.

Huntington's disease is less susceptible to pharmacological treatment. The difficulty here is that GABA is used in all neural networks; drugs that target, mimic or facilitate the actions of GABA will have unwanted and widespread effects throughout the brain. The hyperkinetic symptoms of Huntington's disease, in some cases, can be reduced by the use of dopaminergic antagonists, such as Haloperidol; however, there remains no effective pharmacological therapy for this brain disorder. Likewise, because the neurodegenerative changes in Huntington's disease are more widespread than those seen in Parkinson's disease, deep brain stimulation is unable to provide a viable treatment.

Summary of Section 1.6

The human nervous system consists of millions of cells that form a system of interconnected neural networks; each optimized for the role assigned to them. Some neural networks can be said to be convergent, that is the information processed by them tends to converge on a small population of output neurons; examples are the GABAergic output neurons of the basal ganglia and the Purkinje cells of the cerebellum. Other networks form divergent structures, information is distributed widely throughout the network, examples are the divergence of sensory information from the retina in the visual cortex, and the divergent dopaminergic output from the substantia nigra to the striatum.

The flow of excitatory information in a network is regulated by inhibitory interneurons and the action of neuromodulatory neurotransmitters such as dopamine, serotonin and noradrenalin.

Alterations in the flow of information within neural networks have profound effects on performance and behaviour; such as the symptoms produced by the loss of dopaminergic neurons in Parkinson's disease and the degeneration of striatal GABAergic neurons in Huntington's disease.

1.7 Summary of Chapter 1

This chapter has introduced the key areas required to enable you to understand how neurons communicate. In essence, we can distil this further into three broad concepts.

The first is that neurons store energy in the form of electrically charged molecules called ions. The distribution of these ions on either side of the plasma membrane produces a voltage called the membrane potential. Proteins in the membrane of the neuron, called ion channels, allow ions to pass through the membrane. If a neuron is excited (depolarized) to its firing threshold, it produces an action potential. Once initiated, the action potential rapidly propagates throughout the cell. It is the action potential, made possible by the electrical energy stored as the membrane potential, that allows a cell to send a signal from the site of initiation (usually the axon hillock) to its axon terminals. In other words, the action potential is the cell's own communication system – its own personal intercom!

The second is that most neurons communicate with other neurons by releasing chemical messengers called neurotransmitters – the action potential does not cross the synaptic cleft. Here too, the membrane potential provides the energy that (i) triggers the presynaptic terminal to release neurotransmitter (the entry of extracellular calcium down its concentration and electrical gradients) and (ii) mediates the generation of the synaptic potential in the postsynaptic neuron. The type of neurotransmitter released by the presynaptic terminal and the receptors it binds to on the postsynaptic neuron determines the form and duration of the synaptic potential. Synaptic responses are either excitatory or inhibitory – they either bring the neuron closer to its firing threshold or reduce the likelihood of it firing an action potential.

The third is that neurons are grouped together in specialized units called neural networks. These networks are a function of both their physical structure (the connectivity) and the neurotransmitter systems used. In short, our brains are simply the product of interconnected neural networks!

Learning outcomes for Chapter 1

After studying this chapter, you should be able to:

1.1 Recognize definitions and applications of each of the terms printed in **bold** in the text.

1.2 Describe the principal differences in ion concentrations between the inside and outside of a neuron.

1.3 Describe how concentration gradients and the membrane potential are relevant to understanding the movements of ions across the plasma membrane.

1.4 Explain briefly the role of the sodium–potassium pump in maintaining the resting state of a neuron.

1.5   Explain how an action potential arises in terms of membrane potential, ion channel activation/inactivation and membrane ion permeability.

1.6   Describe how an action potential travels along an axon and what influences its speed.

1.7   Describe the refractory period and explain why it is responsible for the one-way transmission of an action potential along an axon.

1.8   Explain the role of the synapse in the communication and processing of information.

1.9   Describe the sequence of events by which a signal is transmitted across a chemical synapse.

1.10 Explain the difference between an action potential and a synaptic potential.

1.11 Explain the relevance of EPSPs and IPSPs in the initiation of action potentials.

1.12 Explain the difference between an agonist and antagonist.

1.13 Describe the difference between feedforward and feedback inhibition with reference to inhibitory interneurons.

Questions for Chapter 1

Question 1.1   *(Learning outcome 1.2)*

Which of the following descriptions gives an accurate representation of the differences in ion concentration across the neuronal membrane?

Description A

Ion	Concentration	
	Inside cell	Outside cell
sodium	high	low
potassium	high	low
chloride	low	high

Description B

Ion	Concentration	
	Inside cell	Outside cell
sodium	low	high
potassium	high	low
chloride	high	low

Description C

Ion	Concentration	
	Inside cell	Outside cell
sodium	low	high
potassium	high	low
chloride	low	high

Question 1.2   (Learning outcomes 1.3 and 1.4)

Which of the following statement(s) are true?

A   In the resting neuron, the tendency for the concentration gradient of potassium to move potassium ions out of the cell is slightly stronger than the tendency of the resting membrane potential to pull them in.

B   In the resting neuron, as far as sodium ions are concerned, the electrical gradient and concentration gradient act in the same direction.

C   A sodium–potassium pump expels sodium ions from the inside of the neuron and retrieves potassium ions from the outside.

D   Both sodium and potassium ions carry a positive charge.

Question 1.3   (Learning outcome 1.5)

Which of the following statements are true?

A   The initial rising phase of the action potential (depolarization) is due to the opening of voltage-gated sodium channels.

B   The initial rising phase of the action potential is due to the closure of potassium channels.

C   The end of the rising phase of the action potential is due in part to the closure of the sodium channels.

D   The repolarizing phase of the action potential is due to potassium ions being expelled from the cell by the sodium–potassium pump.

E   The hyperpolarization phase of the action potential is due to a delay in closure of voltage-gated potassium channels.

Question 1.4   (Learning outcomes 1.3 and 1.5)

Which of the following statements are true?

A   An EPSP is a move by the local membrane potential away from the resting potential (about −70 mV) to a less negative value.

B   An IPSP is a move of the local membrane potential away from the resting membrane potential to a more negative value.

C   An EPSP could be caused by an opening of receptor-gated channels that allows an increased flow of positive ions into the cell.

D   An EPSP could be caused by an opening of receptor-gated channels that allows an increased flow of negative ions out of the cell.

E   An EPSP could be caused by an opening of receptor-gated channels that allows an increased flow of negative ions into the cell.

F   An IPSP could be caused by an opening of receptor-gated channels that allows an increased flow of positive ions out of the cell.

Question 1.5   (Learning outcome 1.5)

The following is an account of the events underlying the action potential given by a hypothetical SD226 student. Where has the student gone wrong?

'An artificial stimulus is applied to depolarize the membrane. When the threshold is reached, a sudden swing in a positive direction occurs. Voltage-gated sodium channels in the membrane open and sodium ions move into the cell. This is the depolarization phase of the action potential, in other words, a move of membrane potential from a negative value to a less negative value (or more positive value). This move in a positive direction is halted when the sodium channels close and the potassium channels open. The sodium–potassium pump is then responsible for rapidly moving sodium ions out of the cell and this underlies the repolarization phase of the action potential.'

Question 1.6   (Learning outcome 1.6)

Which of the following influence the speed at which an action potential is transmitted along an axon?

A   Whether or not an action potential has recently been generated in the neuron.

B   The diameter of the axon.

C   Whether or not the axon is myelinated.

D   The rate at which sodium is being pumped out of the cell during the passage of the action potential.

E   The length of the axon.

F   The balance of EPSPs and IPSPs that initiated the action potential in the first place.

Question 1.7   (Learning outcome 1.7)

The reason given to explain why an action potential normally travels only one way along an axon concerns the refractory period. However, if an action potential is artificially stimulated at a point somewhere between its two ends, two action potentials can be observed, one moving in each direction away from the point of stimulation. Is it possible to reconcile these two statements in terms of an account involving the refactory period? Explain your answer.

Question 1.8   (Learning outcomes 1.8 and 1.9)

From the list below, select the statement that explains the way in which the electrical synapse differs from the chemical synapse.

A   There is a wider synaptic cleft at electrical synapses.

B   More varied signals can cross the electrical synapse, thereby increasing its capacity to process information.

C   Electrical synapses have a longer synaptic delay than chemical synapses.

D   Transmission across an electrical synapse is much faster than across a chemical synapse, transmission being virtually instantaneous.

Question 1.9   (Learning outcome 1.9)

Identify the numbered parts (1–6) of the chemical synapse represented in Figure 1.31.

Question 1.10   (Learning outcomes 1.8 and 1.9)

Give a brief description of how a signal is transmitted across a chemical synapse.

Question 1.11   (Learning outcome 1.10)

What is the principal difference between an action potential and a synaptic potential?

Question 1.12   (Learning outcome 1.11)

In Figure 1.20 what would be the predicted effect on neuron 4 of action potentials arriving simultaneously from neurons 1 and 3 ?

Question 1.13   (Learning outcome 1.12)

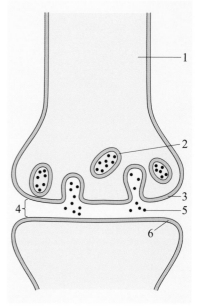

Figure 1.31   For use with Question 1.9.

With reference to the terms agonist and antagonist and the receptor systems involved, how would you describe the following:

(a) nicotine

(b) tetrahydrocannabinol (THC)

(c) Haloperidol

Question 1.14   (Learning outcome 1.13)

Look at Figure 1.25. What would be the consequences for activity in the extensor and flexor muscles of activation of the afferent sensory neuron shown in the figure?

INTERACTING WITH THE ENVIRONMENT: SENSATION AND MOVEMENT

2.1 Introduction

When we think of human brains and what they do, we tend to focus on higher-level processing. We describe someone as 'brainy' if they are, for example, brilliant at mental arithmetic or writing computer programs. In Book 1, Section 1.1.2, you were probably not surprised to read that there was interest in examining Albert Einstein's brain after his death. However, as you went on to read through Chapters 2 and 3 you might have wondered why there was not the same interest in the brain of a talented pianist such as Chopin, for it seems that much of the brain's processing power is used to enable effective physical interaction with the environment – from playing the piano to drinking tea to clambering over slippery rocks.

The great English neurophysiologist Sir Charles Sherrington put it like this:

> I may seem to stress the preoccupation of the brain with muscle. Can we stress too much that preoccupation when any path we trace in the brain leads directly or indirectly to muscle? The brain seems a thoroughfare for nerve action passing on its way to the motor animal. It has been remarked that Life's aim is an act not a thought.

> (Sherrington, 1933)

Central nervous systems, it seems, have evolved to move us around. They have evolved to enable us to explore and make appropriate responses to the environment. A nice illustration of this, which does not require us to peer into the mists of prehistory, is the two-stage life-cycle of some types of sea-squirt. In the larval stage, these creatures swim around to feed. The sea-squirt's primitive nervous system enables it to do this. On reaching maturity however the organism buries its head into a piece of rock and remains there for the rest of its days, feeding simply by filtering seawater. Since it does not have to move, or respond to anything, it doesn't need a nervous system any more and that which it had in the larval stage dissolves away.

We humans may like to think that we use our nervous systems in a rather more varied and extensive manner than the sea-squirt does, but the point remains that, as far as our nervous system goes, our heritage is a movement control system. It seems likely therefore that the way in which we use our brains to negotiate the complexities of our modern social existence is based upon the way we use them to move ourselves around. We will return to this perhaps surprising point later in the chapter when we consider the control of movement.

But before we move around, we need to work out where we are going and why. The development of sophisticated sense organs has provided us with a means of 'sampling' both the external and internal environment. The need for an awareness of the external environment is obvious: we need to know, for example, where the tree is so we don't walk into it and where the stream is if we want to splash in the

water. It may seem less immediately obvious that we also need information from our own bodies (the internal environment). But we do need to know where we are, and whether we are standing or sitting, for example, before we start to move. We will return to the internal environment later in this chapter.

So why do we move? Well, based on the evidence from our senses, we would move out of the way of danger – such as a falling tree or approaching lorry – but whether we play the piano, climb over slippery rocks, drink some tea or run across a meadow will depend on a number of factors to do with our motivation and emotions. (These topics are considered in Book 6.)

In the previous chapter and in Chapter 3 of Book 1, we studied some anatomical and neurochemical details of pathways from senses to brain and from brain to muscles. We have also seen how neurons interconnect to form systems that can process information. In this chapter, we are going to look more closely at some of these systems. In the first half of this chapter we will give an overview of the processing of visual stimuli that allow us to recognize individuals; in the second half we will investigate the means by which skeletal muscles move parts of our bodies when we respond to the person we've just recognized.

2.2   Recognizing your grandmother

Imagine you are walking down a street close to where you live. You see your grandmother walking towards you. You recognize her instantly, even if she is in an unfamiliar location and wearing unfamiliar clothes. Now think what happens if you look at a photograph of your grandparents taken before you were born. The clothes may be strange and old-fashioned, and the hairstyles are probably unfamiliar, but you almost certainly recognize the faces straight away. It is as if there is an essence of that familiar person that shines out through the unfamiliar context.

If you see the face of someone you know well from an unusual angle, perhaps sideways on, you do not consciously have to force yourself to think about what that face would look like from the front, and then try to work out who it is. You just know instantly, and without conscious effort. This lack of effort can make it seem that the task of face recognition is a very easy one. It does not seem hard or complex in the way that playing chess or doing mental arithmetic is hard.

However, we should not be fooled by our intuitions. Face recognition seems easy because we are so very good at it. In fact, it is an incredibly difficult problem.

Consider, by contrast, mental arithmetic. This seems much more difficult than recognizing granny. However, at a computational level, it is really quite simple. A very short computer program can be written that performs arithmetical calculations in a few milliseconds with 100% accuracy. However, when it comes to face recognition, even the best computer system comes nowhere near the performance of a small child – and that child does not even need to try! This means the brain must be doing something very interesting and be exquisitely engineered.

When a task seems effortless, it is not necessarily because the task is actually easy. It is equally likely to be because the brain contains specialized, fast, dedicated circuits to do the relevant computation, and these circuits fire off automatically. They can go wrong, of course. Who has not thought they recognized someone, only to realize with another glance that it is nothing like the person they thought it was. More seriously, the dedicated circuitry can be impaired by brain damage. For

example in Section 4.3.2 of Book 1 you read about the condition called prosopagnosia, where the patient cannot recognize people's faces. There is no problem with their vision in general – the patient can see normally, and tell that what they are seeing is a face; often they can correctly attribute emotion, such as recognizing a happy or sad face. They also remember everything about the person they are looking at as soon as they introduce themselves. The deficit is specifically with recognizing to whom an individual face belongs.

There are even odder deficits related to the brain and vision, such as Capgras' syndrome. With this condition the patient can recognize the face, but believes that although the face *resembles* that of a particular person, such as their father, it is not really their father's face. The emotions that ought to be associated with the patient's father are absent. As a result, Capgras' patients tend to believe that their families have been removed and replaced by impostors who have made themselves look identical to the originals. Interestingly, a patient with Capgras' syndrome accepts their father's voice over the telephone as genuine, but face to face the dissociation between vision and emotion cannot be overridden by the sound of the voice. We are truly very visual animals.

Through a variety of methods, from studying prosopagnosia and Capgras' syndrome to brain imaging, we are beginning to understand the dedicated brain circuits involved in recognizing a familiar face. The next section of this chapter, about the visual system, will be mainly studied using the multimedia package *Exploring the Brain*.

2.3   From eye to brain

The ability to detect a physical stimulus and transform it into a pattern of neural activity is a necessary property of all sensory receptors. The process is called **transduction**. Each sensory receptor responds selectively to specific stimuli. We often say that they are 'tuned' to a particular stimulus modality (also called the *adequate stimulus*). Sensory receptors are categorized according to their adequate stimulus:

- photoreceptors are stimulated by photons of light;
- chemoreceptors are stimulated by chemicals;
- mechanoreceptors are stimulated by mechanical means.

The adequate stimulus causes a change in membrane potential, called the receptor potential (Section 1.5.2, particularly Figure 1.21). This is a *graded* response. The receptor potential changes in size with the size (i.e. intensity) of the stimulus. Many receptor types, such as the photoreceptors in your eyes, can only generate a receptor potential. Action potentials will only appear in neurons further down the visual sensory pathways.

Activity 2.1

You should now study the Vision section of the multimedia package *Exploring the Brain*. You have already studied the basic anatomy of the visual pathways and some of the functions of its components in Book 1, Chapters 3 and 4. It may be advantageous to have another look at those chapters as you study the Vision section.

From your study of the Vision section of the multimedia package *Exploring the Brain*, you should now have an understanding of the ways in which the characteristics of the visual scene are coded and conveyed to the brain. It shows that the photoreceptors of the retina convert the patterns of light from the visual scene into a neural image. But it is not this neural image that is conveyed along the visual pathways to the brain's visual cortex. Instead, using different streams or pathways for different kinds of information, the eye 'tells' the brain about particular aspects of the scene, such as colour, shape and movement.

Figure 2.1 shows the basic structure of the human eye. Figure 2.2 is a schematic cross-section of the retina of a vertebrate. The photoreceptors are the **rods** and **cones**. Cone activity underlies colour vision. The interconnected cells of the plexiform layers thereafter allow for the initial processing of the neural image captured by the photoreceptors. Except at the fovea, which consists of cones at a very high density, photoreceptors converge onto bipolar cells. The result of the retinal processing is that the **retinal ganglion cells**, the first cells in the visual pathway to show an action potential, have complex, circular receptive fields. In other words they are connected, via neurons in the plexiform layers, to photoreceptors that between them respond to light from a circular area of the visual field. The retinal ganglion cells have a steady rate of firing in the absence of any change in the visual stimulation. (This, of course, does not happen very often – except in experiments!) They change their firing rate (either increasing it or decreasing it) only if there is visual change somewhere within their receptive field. Figure 2.3 shows how stimulating any photoreceptor whose output contributes to the centre of the retinal ganglion cell's receptive field will have the opposite effect on the retinal ganglion cell's firing pattern to stimulating a photoreceptor whose output contributes to the annular periphery of the retinal ganglion cell's receptive field. Note how the axons of the retinal ganglion cells lie alongside one another to form the optic nerve (Figure 2.2).

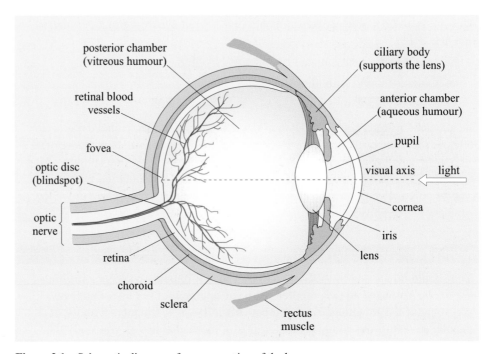

Figure 2.1   Schematic diagram of a cross-section of the human eye.

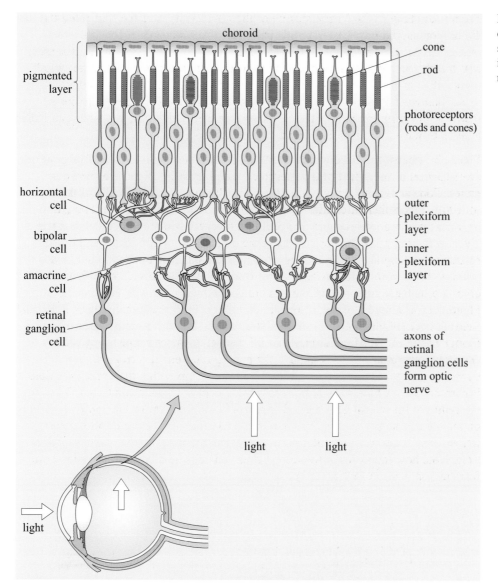

Figure 2.2 Schematic cross-section of the retina of a vertebrate. (Insert shows a diagram of the human eye and indicates the relationship between the retina and incoming light.)

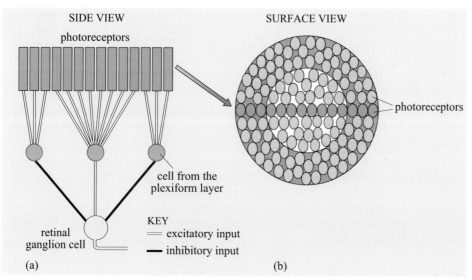

Figure 2.3 (a) Receptors in the receptive field send information to the retinal ganglion cell. (b) Diagram showing the receptive field of the retinal ganglion cell in (a).

The Vision section of the multimedia package *Exploring the Brain* indicates that there are different types of retinal ganglion cell. The different types encode different aspects of the visual stimuli. This is achieved partly by the types of receptor from which they receive input and partly by the ways in which these inputs are 'wired together'.

The pathways from eye to brain are shown in Figure 2.4, together with the defects produced by three lesions made before, after, and at the **optic chiasma**. All retinal ganglion cells synapse in the **lateral geniculate nucleus (LGN) in the thalamus.** There are six layers of neurons in the LGN. Each layer receives input from just one eye. Neurons in the two ventral layers have large cell bodies and are known as **magnocellular** layers (from the Latin *magnus*, large); the four dorsal layers are called the **parvocellular** layers (from the Latin *parvus*, small). Projections from the retina to the magnocellular and parvocellular layers of the lateral geniculate nuclei are given in Figure 2.5a. The projections retain a precisely ordered pattern, known as **retinotopic** mapping. This mapping is retained in the areas in the occipital lobes (the primary visual cortex) that receive input from the eyes (Figure 2.5b). Figure 2.6a gives a schematic summary of the anatomical pathways through the visual cortex. Figure 2.6b is a repeat of the schematic diagram of retinal inputs that was in Book 1, Section 4.4.2 (Figure 4.14). From this you can see that the magnocellular pathway feeds through to the dorsal stream and the parvocellular pathway feeds through to the ventral stream.

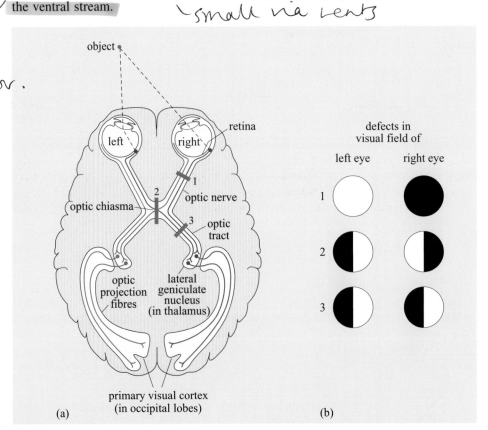

(a)

(b)

Figure 2.4   (a) Map of the positions of lesions at different points in the visual pathway. (b) Defects in the visual field produced by lesions at the different levels shown in (a). Cutting the optic nerve (1) produces complete loss of vision in the right eye. Cutting the optic chiasma (2) produces a complete loss of the temporal visual field in each eye. The field losses do not overlap. Cutting the optic tract (3) causes a complete loss of vision in both eyes in the contralateral visual fields.

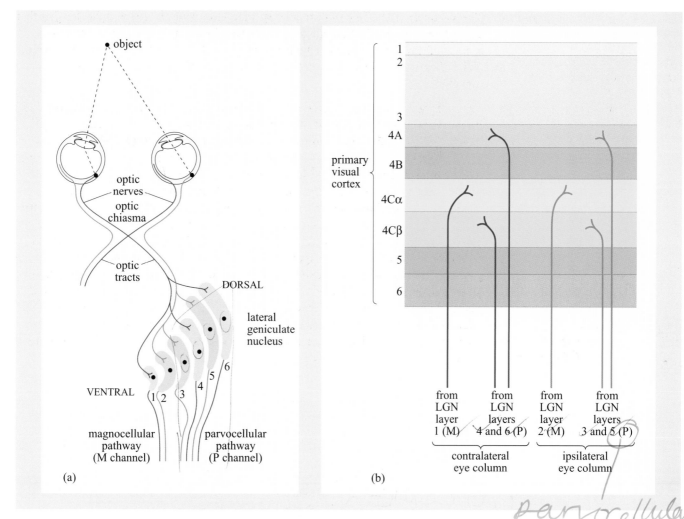

Figure 2.5   (a) Magnocellular (M) and parvocellular (P) pathways through the lateral geniculate nucleus to the visual cortex. The individual layers of the LGN are coloured to indicate whether their output is from the contralateral (blue) or ipsilateral (green) eye. (b) LGN axons from different eyes and from different layers arrive in different sublayers or in different zones of the primary visual cortex.

parvocellular

small

parvo-
parvo- small
portion

Figure 2.6 (a) Schematic summary of anatomical pathways from the retina to the visual cortex. (b) Dorsal, ventral and subcortical visual processing streams, shown schematically. Abbreviations: LGN is the lateral geniculate nucleus, SC is the superior colliculus. Both the LGN and the pulvinar nucleus are thalamic structures.

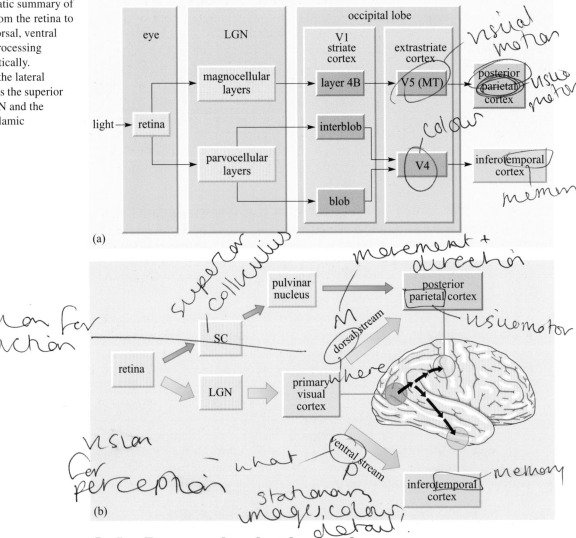

2.4 Processing in the brain

Before continuing with the story of the processing of information from the eyes, we should note that about 10% of the axons leaving the retina lead to structures in the midbrain such as the superior colliculus. This small non-cortical pathway represents a low-level visual system, which may be used in certain fast behaviours such as startle reflexes and the accurate movement of a bat or racquet to intercept a rapidly moving ball in games such as cricket or tennis. These rapid responses are possible because the route from retina to superior colliculus is direct and fast, the superior colliculus receives the visual information very quickly. In addition, the superior colliculus has direct connections (not shown in Figure 2.6b) to the motor systems controlling eye movements, reaching and so forth. It is this non-cortical pathway which is thought to be spared in the disorder known as blindsight, which you met in Book 1, Section 1.1.6 and Chapter 4. Patients with blindsight report no experience of seeing anything, but demonstrate by the way they move that information from the eyes is available to guide their movements. The characteristic damage in blindsight is to area V1 striate cortex in the occipital lobe.

So there are different pathways in the visual system from and to different areas, and they do different things. The cortical pathway was investigated further by

recording from single cells in these different areas. It was found that the neurons in the primary visual cortex (V1) are of several types, and respond in more complex ways than the neurons in the retina or lateral geniculate nucleus. For example some neurons respond maximally when an edge appears in their receptive field, while others respond only when there is movement, colour or a particular shape. The receptive fields of these neurons in the cortex are not all circular, but come in various shapes and sizes. The discovery that there were different distributions of specialization was the trigger that led to the hypothesis that the magnocellular and parvocellular pathways were designed to do different things. The magnocellular pathway is, according to this hypothesis, concerned with motion and spatial location, whereas the parvocellular pathway, drawing as it does on information about colour and form, is concerned with object recognition and discrimination.

- In Book 1, Section 4.4.2 we stated that the speed of transmission differs in the magnocellular and parvocellular pathways, and in Section 2.4.3 of Book 1 and Section 1.3.3 of this book there has been some discussion of transmission speeds in differently sized axons. Which pathway do you think has the more rapid transmission? Try to work out the probable answer. (Remember that structure and function are usually related.)

- The magnocellular pathway analyses motion, which needs to be done rather quickly; it also has cells with thick axons. The thick axons conduct more rapidly than thin axons. You should have deduced that the magnocellular pathway has the more rapid transmission speed, or you may have remembered from Book 1, Table 4.1b.

The magnocellular and parvocellular pathways have become popularly known as the 'where?' and 'what?' systems respectively.

- In terms of the two streams of information that pass through the cortex (the dorsal and ventral streams), which is the 'where?' system?

- The 'where?' system is the dorsal stream which has its input from the dorsal magnocellular layers of the lateral geniculate nucleus and terminates in the posterior parietal cortex.

There is additional evidence that the two streams actually perform these different functions.

- What kinds of evidence or experiments might be used to demonstrate that the two visual processing streams really do have the 'where?' and 'what?' functions?

- There are several possibilities. One is brain imaging. The hypothesis predicts that there will be greater activation in the parietal pathway when a participant is doing a task that involves the detection of motion or spatial relations, and greater activation in the temporal pathway in a task involving colour or complex object recognition. Another source of possible evidence comes from brain damage. The hypothesis predicts that different types of visual impairment will follow from parietal and temporal brain damage.

2.4.1 Brain imaging

Semir Zeki and his colleagues in London (Zeki *et al.*, 1991) set out to use PET scanning directly to test the hypothesis that the parietal (dorsal) stream was specialized for motion and the temporal (ventral) stream was specialized for colour.

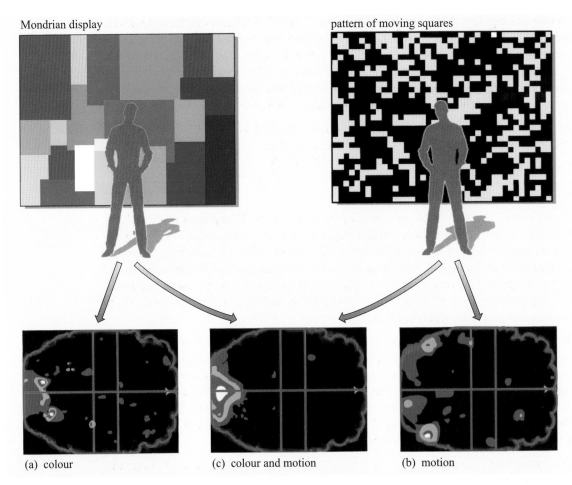

Mondrian display

pattern of moving squares

(a) colour   (c) colour and motion   (b) motion

Figure 2.7   Regions of increased cerebral blood flow in the human brain when the participant views (a) a multicoloured Mondrian display and (b) a pattern of moving squares. Highest increases are shown in white, red and yellow. The regions of high cerebral blood flow are indicated in horizontal slices through the cerebral cortex. Note that there is a difference in location between the area activated by the colour stimulus (V4) and the one activated by the motion stimulus (V5). The primary visual cortex (V1) shown in (c) was active in all cases.

They set up experiments where the participants had to look at abstract scenes containing edges but no recognizable objects, rather like the works of the painter Mondrian. These scenes could be colourful or monochrome grey. They could also be still or contain moving squares. The experimenters compared brain activity when the scenes were multicoloured versus monochrome, and moving versus still.

The primary visual cortex (V1) was highly active in all cases (Figure 2.7c). However, motion produced a sharp increase in activation in V5 (also called the middle temporal (MT) area), but not V4 (Figure 2.7b), whereas the addition of colour produced a sharp increase in V4 but not V5 (Figure 2.7a). The results could not be clearer or more elegant: V4 is involved in colour vision, and V5 in the perception of movement.

2.4.2   Brain damage

As you know, the visual system has specialized subsystems. This has implications for what happens when the brain is damaged. When brain damage occurs it is usually messy, damaging or partly damaging many different areas, and perhaps damaging one side more than the other. However, from time to time, chance produces a patient with very specific and localized damage. When damage of this nature occurs to the visual

system, the results are very striking. The loss of visual function is seldom general; that is to say, the patient is not just a little worse at all visual tasks. Instead, they perform at normal levels on some tasks, and with a great loss of ability on others. This is further evidence for specialization within the visual system. In this section we are only going to consider one type of impairment, the one that relates specifically to the task we are particularly concerned with understanding: recognizing granny.

The term **agnosia** (from the Greek *agnoia*, ignorance) was coined by Freud in 1891 to refer to a family of conditions in which the patient loses the ability to recognize objects. There are several different types of agnosia, but they all share the common feature in that the patient sees an object, and can clearly perceive the individual features that it has, but cannot judge what it is.

A stroke patient called H.J.A. was studied by Riddoch and Humphreys (1987). H.J.A. had suffered a blockage of a cerebral artery, and so had lost the blood supply to part of the back of his brain (Book 1, Box 3.4). Since the incident, patient H.J.A. had become profoundly impaired at all tasks to do with visual recognition, namely recognizing faces, objects, written words, and colours. For example, when presented with a paintbrush he said, 'it appears to be two things close together but obviously it is one thing or you would have told me.'

Studies of this patient showed that his knowledge of objects was unimpaired; he could answer questions about what paintbrushes are like as well as ever. He had no problem recognizing objects by touch or sound. His vision had been disturbed by his injury, but not seriously so. This is demonstrated by the fact that he could copy a drawing extremely well. It is clear from his responses that H.J.A. could access information about the parts of things he was looking at, but had problems perceiving the way they went together to make a whole, distinctive object.

The damage characteristic of this type of agnosia is in V4 and the areas of temporal cortex surrounding it.

◆   What does agnosia suggest about the function of the temporal visual pathway?

◆   It suggests that the temporal visual pathway serves to identify objects by seeing 'the whole' and somehow mapping this to our stored knowledge of various types of objects.

Summary of Section 2.4

A small proportion of the visual output from the retina goes to the superior colliculi. The pathway via the superior colliculi is used to guide fast behaviour, such as hitting a tennis ball. Individuals with blindsight have this pathway intact but have damage to the occipital lobe.

The major pathways in the primary visual cortex are the parietal pathway from the magnocellular layers and the temporal pathway from the parvocellular layers.

Information from brain imaging and from brain-damaged individuals confirms that the parietal stream is concerned with motion and spatial location, whereas the temporal stream is concerned with object recognition.

2.5   A familiar face?

We began this chapter by asking what happens in the brain when you recognize the face of your grandmother. Interest in face perception was sparked off in the 1970s,

when it was discovered that in the monkey there are neurons in the temporal lobe that fire off rapidly in response to the presentation of a face (of a human or another monkey). These cells do not respond so strongly to a paw or to an inanimate object of similar size and shape to a face such as a square or circle (Figure 2.8) or to an image made from a jumble of parts of faces. This last demonstration is particularly important, since the jumbled image had all the same elements as a face, but in a different configuration. This means that the cells are specially tuned to the whole face, not to the parts that make it up.

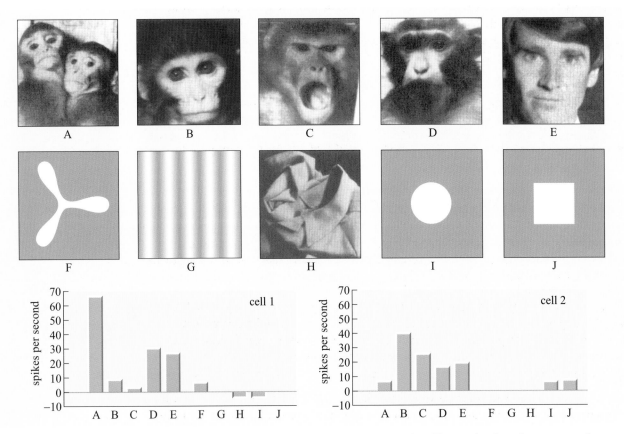

Figure 2.8   Response of face cells in the superior temporal sulcus of the macaque monkey. The graphs show the response of two cells to the ten stimuli (labelled A–J). Both cells responded vigorously to many of the facial stimuli. However, when the animal looked at the objects, there was either no change in activity or, in some cases, the cells were actually inhibited relative to the baseline. The firing rate data are plotted as a change from baseline activity for that cell when no stimulus was presented. (Adapted from Baylis *et al.*, 1985)

Is this evidence that the primate brain, including perhaps our own, contains a special module just for recognizing faces? The hypothesis makes some evolutionary sense. It is imperative for all primates to recognize quickly other individuals around them, to know with whom they are dealing and what sort of behaviour is appropriate. This is as true for us as it is for monkeys and apes. However, evolutionary plausibility is one thing; but is there direct evidence for a special face recognition module in the brain?

Many studies of face recognition have been carried out. Face recognition is fast. Brain-imaging studies have shown that a cortical area on the fusiform gyrus is much more strongly activated when looking at faces than when looking at words, animals, objects, or the backs of human heads. This area, which has become known as the **fusiform face area (FFA)**, is on the margin of the temporal lobe (see Book 1, Figure 4.20), and corresponds to the location of the face-specific neurons identified

in the monkey brain. Most strikingly, there are patients with damage in this region who lose their ability to recognize faces.

◈   What is the name for this syndrome?

◆   This syndrome is called prosopagnosia (Section 2.2).

As with other agnosias, it is not a loss of general knowledge or intellectual ability, since patients can recognize the voices of, and talk knowledgeably about, the people whose faces they cannot recognize. They simply cannot tell who someone is from seeing their face alone. Prosopagnosia is not necessarily accompanied by agnosia relating to other types of object. There is also at least one patient with agnosia who is severely impaired on reading and object recognition, but absolutely fine when it comes to recognizing faces (Moscovitch *et al.*, 1997).

◈   What would you infer about pathways involved in face and other object processing from the above data?

◆   You would infer that faces are processed in a different place in the brain from other objects.

◈   It is often concluded that the FFA has evolved as a specialized face detection module. Is that the only possible explanation of the data?

◆   It is one interpretation. Another interpretation is that the FFA is a specialized module for making fine discriminations between individuals or objects belonging to the same category.

Most of the other object recognition tasks mentioned above involved saying only to which category something belonged (horse, arm, iron, etc.), and the differences between these different objects are large. In face recognition, we are dealing with small differences between individuals within the same category. It could be that the FFA is for within-category individuation in general, rather than for faces as such.

We have, then, two interpretations of the activity of the FFA: one in which it is for all types of individual discrimination, and one in which it is dedicated to individual faces.

◈   How might you test between these two interpretations?

◆   You would need to devise a task where the participants were able to individuate between many different, similar individuals or objects of the same general category. You would predict that the FFA would be active in such tasks. You would also predict that prosopagnosic patients would have problems with such tasks.

Both of these predictions have been investigated. Isabel Gauthier and her colleagues, using functional MRI scanning, have conducted studies with participants who are experts in recognizing either birds or cars, (Gauthier *et al.*, 2000). The participants looked at pictures of different types of cars, or of birds or of faces on a screen, and tried to identify them. The investigators found that for all the participants, faces strongly activated the FFA in the right hemisphere. However:

•   for the bird experts, pictures of birds activated the FFA more than did pictures of cars;

•   for the car experts, pictures of cars activated the FFA more strongly than did pictures of birds.

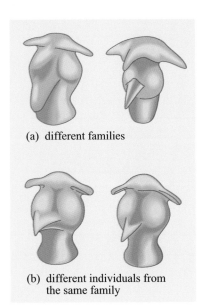

(a) different families

(b) different individuals from the same family

Figure 2.9 Greebles: (a) two individuals from different families; (b) two individuals from the same family.

The same team have also conducted functional MRI experiments with a set of invented stimuli known as 'greebles' (Figure 2.9). Greebles are shapes which vary subtly from one another. With practice, you can learn to recognize individual greebles and put them into 'families' that show strong resemblances. The investigators trained the participants over a number of sessions until they could recognize individual greebles and quickly assign them to families. They showed that the activation of the right FFA was not particularly great in the early sessions. However, as the participants became more expert, the right FFA became more and more strongly activated when looking at greebles. After eight training sessions, the right FFA responded nearly (but not quite) as strongly to greebles as to faces.

◆ What is the implication of the greebles experiment and the bird and car expert studies for the function of the FFA?

◆ It implies that the FFA is not so much dedicated to face recognition, as used for making judgements about the individual identity of objects which we are expert at discriminating, regardless of whether those objects are faces or not. For this reason, Gauthier has suggested that 'FFA' would be better taken to mean 'flexible fusiform area' than 'fusiform face area'!

Another source of evidence comes from prosopagnosia. If the FFA is more generally involved in object recognition than just faces, then prosopagnosic patients should show impairments on all types of expert discrimination, not just face recognition. It is true that many prosopagnosics have a broader agnosia, but of course this may be because the brain damage is broader than just the FFA (after all, nature is rarely a neat experimenter). One well-known prosopagnosic patient had been a keen birdwatcher before the accident, but lost the ability to recognize bird species after the accident. Others, however, show an opposite pattern, such as retaining the ability to discriminate many different types of car but not able to recognize faces. One patient even became a shepherd after his accident, and became adept at recognizing his individual sheep, despite his inability to recognize the individual faces of his friends and family.

◆ Do you think the FFA is specialized for face recognition, or has it got a more general function?

◆ The answer is not totally clear. The greeble experiment and the car and bird expert studies support a general interpretation, but evidence from face-specific neurons in the monkey brain and patients with prosopagnosia seems to point the other way. Perhaps a compromise is possible; the FFA is usually used to process faces, which are one of the most significant kinds of stimuli in the human environment, but it can be recruited to other tasks when individuals become particularly interested or expert in them. This would be an example of neural plasticity (Book 3, Section 3.3.2).

Summary of Section 2.5

Neurons in the temporal lobe of monkeys seem to fire in response to faces. In humans, damage to a similar area on the margins of the temporal lobe, the fusiform face area (FFA), results in prosopagnosia. However other evidence, such as the categorization of cars, birds and greebles, suggests that the FFA might not be a specialist area for face recognition, being equally capable of distinguishing between very similar classes of object.

2.6   Introduction to the control of movement

In this chapter, we have gradually built up a picture of how you might recognize – quickly and effortlessly – the face of your grandmother. The visual pathway from eye to brain has multiple stages and, at each stage, more complex features are extracted from the visual scene and fed forwards to the next stage. The cells at the highest stages of processing are specialized for recognizing quite complex and specific objects, such as faces. When the criteria for 'face-like' are met, those cells suddenly fire off, which might explain the sudden way a face, especially a familiar one, 'pops out' of the background as you suddenly recognize it.

Of course, recognition requires awareness. We do not always recognize a familiar face. Who has not faced the embarrassing situation of meeting a friend who claims that you ignored them last week? 'You walked right by me and never said hello!' Instead of muttering an apology you can explain that your lapse was caused by *inattentional blindness* and then demonstrate the strength of this phenomenon by recounting the experiments involving gorillas at basketball games and construction workers asking directions (Book 1, Section 4.5.3).

So now with this in mind, let us return in our imagination to the street where a woman is walking towards us. You recognize her as your granny and you wave to her. Let's consider what this involves. In your earlier studies (Book 1, Section 4.4.2), you were introduced to the idea of two visual brains working together. The ventral stream, with the FFA designated as an *essential node*, needs to be intact to enable you to recognize your granny and to decide how to respond. But your non-conscious dorsal stream is involved in the implementation of these decisions. 'Waving' seems to be such a simple action to control. However, with all the possible links between cortical and subcortical pathways, the control of even an apparently simple activity is complex. So we shall begin our introduction to the control of movement by looking at something that *is* comparatively well understood and straightforward: the basic mechanisms of muscle control.

We have already touched on some of the basic mechanisms involved in movement (particularly in Book 1, Chapter 3), as well as the different levels (or layers) of control. One fundamental dichotomy that has been addressed is the difference between the 'housekeeping' muscle movements involved in activities such as digestion and pumping blood around the body, and the muscle movements involved in moving the skeleton around.

◆   What are the names and functions of the three types of muscle?

◆   Skeletal muscle moves the limbs, cardiac muscle keeps the heart beating, and smooth muscle controls the flow of blood through blood vessels and food through the gut (Book 1, Section 1.3.2).

◆   Which division of the nervous system is involved in 'housekeeping' activities?

◆   The autonomic nervous system (Book 1, Section 2.3.1).

The rest of this chapter will concern itself with the direct control of skeletal muscle by the CNS. This is what Sherrington called 'the final common pathway'. We will try to avoid a totally reductionist approach because it is important not to lose sight of the bigger picture. For example one of the most straightforward of motor responses, the muscle stretch reflex, was described in Book 1, Section 3.3.2.

Towards the end of that section we stated that the nociceptive (or withdrawal) reflex is organized at the same level as the stretch reflex in the CNS.

◆   At what level in the CNS are these responses organized?

◆   These responses are organized at the level of the spinal cord.

◆   In Book 1, Section 3.3.2, it was suggested that the nociceptive response might be given in response to being pricked by a rose thorn. In what way would you modify Figure 2.10a to enable you to show this nociceptive reflex response?

◆   The site of the stimulation must be altered, as shown in Figure 2.10b.

However, the reflex withdrawal from an unpleasant stimulus is unlikely to be the only consequence of prickling yourself on a thorn. You soon experience some level of pain or discomfort, you might examine your skin and you may make some comment (or even utter an expletive).

◆   How can the stimulus of the thorn piercing the skin lead to activation of other parts of the CNS, and the ANS, as well as activation of the muscle reflex?

◆   The sensory afferent neuron will feed information into ascending pathways. For example, Book 1, Section 3.4.6 states that there are pathways to the brain that are also activated when you prick your thumb or sustain any other kind of tissue damage, and that the sensation of pain occurs when these sensory inputs are processed in the brain. Subsequently, descending pathways to the ANS can become active.

◆   Name the pathway (in Figure 2.11) that conveys sensation from the pierced skin.

◆   The sensation is conveyed by activity occurring in the anterolateral system.

Figure 2.10   (a) The neuronal pathways involved in a muscle stretch reflex. The afferent neuron is labelled 1, the efferent neurons are labelled 2, 3 and 5 and the interneuron is labelled 4. (b) The nociceptive reflex pathway to being pricked on the back of the hand by a rose thorn. Note that in this diagram the ending of the afferent sensory neuron is embedded in the back of the hand as opposed to in the muscle but the neuronal connections are similar to those shown in (a).

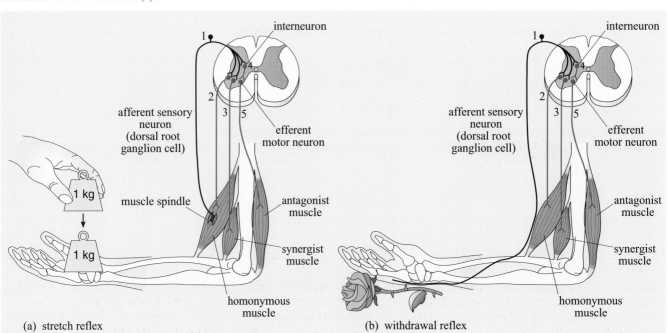

(a) stretch reflex   (b) withdrawal reflex

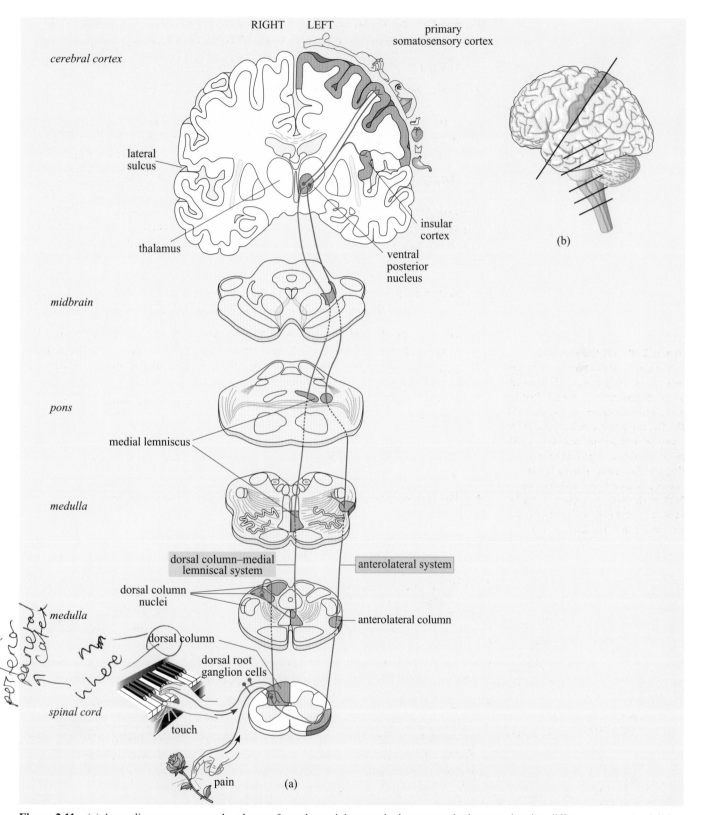

Figure 2.11   (a) Ascending sensory neural pathways from the periphery to the human cerebral cortex showing different sensory modalities. The pathway for touch, the dorsal column–medial lemniscal system (DCMLS), is indicated in red and that for temperature and noxious stimuli (such as pain), the anterolateral system (ALS), is indicated in purple. Note that the pathways cross-over to the contralateral side at different anatomical levels, the spinal cord for the ALS and the medulla for the DCMLS. (b) The locations of the various cross-sections shown in (a) taken through the spinal cord and brain.

Having reminded ourselves that motor responses organized at the spinal level do not work in total isolation from the rest of the CNS, we will now take a reductionist approach as we begin by studying the effectors of this system – the skeletal muscles.

2.7   Skeletal muscles

Muscles produce movement. Typically, a skeletal muscle is attached by a tendon to a bone, spans one or more joints, and is then attached by another tendon to another bone. This is why we describe muscles as *crossing* joints. When a muscle receives a signal from the CNS, it attempts to contract (i.e. to pull its two ends closer together) or get shorter. When a muscle shortens it produces movement (Figure 2.12). If the muscle fails to shorten, it instead develops increased tension and we say that the muscle is working isometrically.

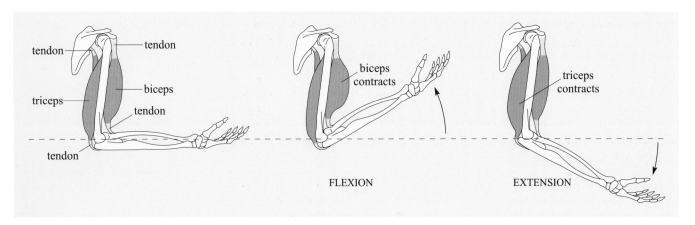

Figure 2.12   Biceps and triceps respectively flex and extend the elbow joint – they form an antagonistic pair of muscles. Such a pair of muscles is the minimum requirement for moving a joint because muscles can only contract actively – they cannot lengthen actively. Joints like the shoulder and hip, which have more freedom of movement than a hinge joint such as the elbow or knee, require more muscles adequately to control their movement.

The action of muscles is to contract. They cannot actively lengthen. Therefore in the simplest type of joint, a hinge-type joint such as the elbow, there must be at least two muscles:

- one muscle opens (extends) the hinge when it shortens;
- one muscle closes (flexes) the hinge when it shortens.

In the elbow, these two muscles are called triceps (extension) and biceps (flexion). Such a group of two muscles is said to form an antagonistic pair. In a sense, this label is a bit misleading. It is true that these two muscles have opposing actions but, rather than 'antagonizing' one another, they have in fact to work synergistically (i.e. together) to bring about the desired action at the joint. For example, if the aim is to flex the elbow (i.e. bring the hand towards the shoulder), biceps must contract and triceps must not contract; a muscle that is not contracting is said to be relaxed.

Sometimes, however, both muscles in an antagonistic pair are found to be contracting at the same time. This **co-contraction** has the effect of stiffening the joint, making it more difficult to move. Note that in this case both the muscles are contracting isometrically, this means that instead of getting shorter they are developing increased tension. Some degree of co-contraction is often essential.

◆   Give an example of a situation where co-contraction of muscles is necessary.

◆   In Book 1, Section 3.3.2 you read about the co-contraction of synergistic muscles that enabled the hand to remain steady whilst extra weights were added. You might have thought of other everyday examples. For example, when writing

a letter, we stiffen the elbow (and shoulder) joints to help the hand move slowly and precisely. When using an electric sander, we also stiffen the joints of the arm to prevent the sander veering off on its own course and scratching the grain of the wood.

In general, whether the aim is to make a joint move, or make it difficult to move, all of the muscles which pass over the joint need to cooperate. The job of ensuring cooperation falls to the movement control system, which is in the CNS. We will start by looking at how the CNS controls an individual muscle, and then at how it coordinates the action of the various muscles passing over (crossing) a single joint. We'll then go on to look at the control of the more complex movements which we all make everyday, which require the coordinated action of many joints.

2.7.1   Control of a single muscle

The CNS causes a muscle to contract by sending action potentials along motor neurons called **alpha motor neurons**. These neurons have their cell bodies in the ventral horn of the spinal cord (or in the brainstem for muscles of the head). Their axons can be traced from the spinal cord via the ventral roots and then along progressively smaller branches of peripheral nerves until they reach the muscle that they innervate. Here, each axon branches extensively, synapsing with a large number of cells in a muscle. Although one alpha motor neuron connects to many muscle cells, the converse is not the case. Normally, each muscle cell is innervated by only one motor neuron.

The muscle's cells are called **muscle fibres**. Like neurons they are *excitable* cells, able to produce action potentials. The motor neuron's axon terminal forms a synapse with the muscle fibre. This synapse is called the **neuromuscular junction**. An action potential arriving at the presynaptic terminal triggers the release of the neurotransmitter acetylcholine (ACh). Neuromuscular junctions are large compared to synapses between neurons and they are relatively easier to access for experimental purposes. So most of the initial work elucidating the properties of chemical synapses was done using the neuromuscular junction. The arrival of the action potential at the neuromuscular junction triggers the opening of the Ca^{2+} ion channels. The entry of Ca^{2+} ions enables the release of ACh from the vesicles. ACh diffuses across the gap and attaches to receptors on the muscle fibre.

◈   What is the name of these receptors?

◆   They are called nicotinic receptors (Section 1.4.4 and Box 1.2).

◈   What is the effect on the muscle fibres of the ACh attaching to the nicotinic receptors?

◆   The muscle is excited.

◈   What kind of potential is observed at the postsynaptic membrane of the neuromuscular junction?

◆   An excitatory postsynaptic potential (EPSP).

◆ In what way does the neural input to the muscle fibre differ from the neural input to neurons?

◆ Each muscle fibre is innervated by one motor neuron only. In most cases, the neural inputs to neurons number in the hundreds or thousands. These multiple inputs are integrated at the axon hillock. There is no equivalent of an axon hillock in a muscle fibre.

The postsynaptic membrane of the neuromuscular junction is called a *motor end plate* – the potential is therefore known as the motor end plate potential. When a motor neuron fires, releasing molecules of ACh that attach to nicotinic receptors, an action potential is always produced in the muscle fibre. Whilst molecules of ACh occupy nicotinic receptors the muscle fibre remains depolarized, continuing to produce action potentials.

◆ What terminates this activity?

◆ An enzyme called acetylcholinesterase (AChE) degrades ACh at the motor end plate (Section 1.4.4 and Box 1.2).

So, the motor neuron's action potential reaches the muscle and gives rise to an action potential in all the muscle fibres that it innervates. The action potential causes the muscle fibres to contract briefly, or **twitch**.

◆ Is it possible to get half the muscle fibres innervated by one alpha motor neuron to twitch?

◆ No, it is not possible for a motor neuron to get just half of the muscle fibres it innervates to twitch. There are only two options: a twitch in all of the fibres or a twitch in none of them.

For this reason an alpha motor neuron and the muscle fibres it innervates are called a **motor unit** (Figure 2.13). The term was first used by Charles Sherrington. The number of fibres in a motor unit varies both within and between muscles. Small muscles such as those of the hand that produce relatively small forces and are involved in fine control might have some motor units comprising just 10 muscle fibres, but will have other motor units with up to about 100 muscle fibres. Such a muscle might have about 100 motor units in all. Large muscles such as biceps may have motor units with between 100 and 1000 muscle fibres, and nearly 1000 motor units in all. Note that the muscle fibres of an individual motor unit are typically quite widely distributed within the muscle.

A single twitch of one motor unit is the smallest possible unit of motor activity. A twitch is about one-tenth of a second (0.1 s or 100 milliseconds) in duration. These extremely brief twitches are tiny and are the building blocks of all our movements, all of our behaviour. Everything we do is made up of them. What we now need to understand is how the CNS manages to produce purposeful and controlled movement, such as waving, playing the piano or clambering over slippery rocks, just by combining huge numbers of these tiny contractile events.

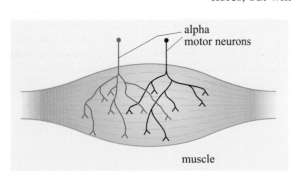

Figure 2.13   An alpha motor neuron branches when it reaches the muscle it innervates and synapses with many individual muscle fibres. The neuron together with the muscle fibres it innervates is termed a motor unit.

2.7.2   How the CNS produces sustained muscle contraction

An action potential is a very fast event, it lasts about 2 milliseconds in a muscle fibre. We have already noted that the twitch it produces is much longer in duration, about fifty times as long, which is about 100 ms or more (Figure 2.14). But this is still an extremely brief event. It lasts one-tenth of a second, too short an interval of time to appreciate easily. The muscle contractions required for purposeful movement are of much longer duration than this. The CNS produces these relatively long-duration contractions by using many motor units together. To produce a continuous contraction, such as that required to hold up an object in a certain position, each of these units twitches at a roughly constant rate, such as between 10 and 20 times a second. But each unit is set to a slightly different rate. The result is that in general they all fire at different times, in other words they fire asynchronously. In the muscle as a whole, all of the individual twitches are summed together to produce a sustained and approximately continuous contraction.

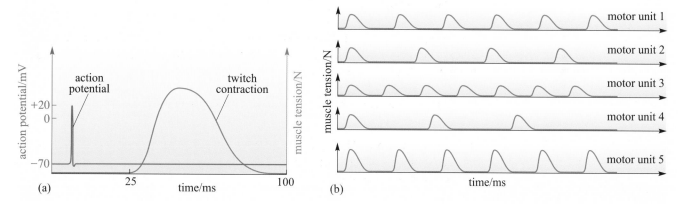

In certain conditions, for example Parkinson's disease, the CNS can lose this ability to produce fully asynchronous firing of the motor units and a degree of synchronicity begins to emerge. This can be extremely debilitating because, rather than producing continuous levels of contraction, it produces a wobble or tremor (Section 1.6.4). The most obvious sign of this is a rhythmic shaking of the hands, but as the disease progresses it can take over the whole body. You may have experienced tremor yourself if you've ever carried a heavy suitcase or similar for quite a long time and then tried to drink a cup of tea. You may have been unable to hold the cup steady because your arm was shaking. Like any other, this tremor is due to (partially) synchronous firing of motor units, caused in this case by fatigue. This example demonstrates how important an asynchronous firing pattern is. Happily, as you recover from your exertions, the tremor goes away.

Figure 2.14   (a) The action potential of the muscle fibre is of much shorter duration than the twitch contraction that it produces. (b) A number of motor units all firing at different frequencies produce a near-random firing pattern known as asynchronous firing. The result at the level of the muscle as a whole is an approximately continuous contraction. Note: N stands for newton, a unit of force.

2.7.3   How the CNS changes the strength of muscle contraction

One of the things that we require of our muscles is that they can produce a wide range of levels of continuous contractile force. This enables us, for example, to hold a cup of tea by the saucer without spilling the contents (something that requires a small contractile force) and to lift a large heavy saucepan of boiled potatoes and drain them without mishap (something that requires a large contractile force).

◆ From what you have read about the way that neurons work, suggest how it is possible to alter the strength of contraction in your muscles.

◆ The CNS has two ways of increasing the contractile force being produced by a muscle:

• It can recruit (start using) more motor units. From the discussion so far it should be intuitively apparent that using more motor units would increase the overall contractile force.

• It can increase the firing frequency of the motor neurons that are already active. The effect of increasing the action potential firing rate on neurotransmitter release was discussed in Section 1.5.2, so from that you might have guessed that contractile force could be increased in this way.

In fact, when the firing frequency of a motor unit increases sufficiently, one action potential follows another so quickly that the second occurs during the twitch contraction produced by the first. This results in the two twitch contractions combining (Figure 2.15).

Figure 2.15 (a) Well-spaced action potentials produce discrete twitches (the first is all over before the second starts). (b) If a second action potential occurs before the first twitch is complete, the second twitch is larger than normal. Summation is said to have occurred. Note: this can only happen because the twitch contraction is so much longer in duration than the action potential. (c) Repeated firing at high frequency (for example 35 events per second or 35 hertz, usually abbreviated 35 Hz) produces progressive summation of contractile force until a maximum contraction is reached.

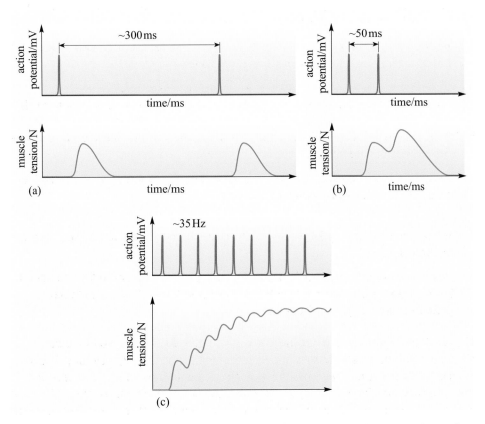

In practice, the CNS uses both recruitment (and decruitment) of motor units and adjustment of the firing rate in order to produce the large range of contractile forces required. This said, in smaller muscles the adjustment of firing rate is the more important mechanism, whereas in larger muscles recruitment and decruitment is favoured.

There are several other subtleties surrounding the recruitment of motor units because the motor units in a muscle are not all the same. First of all, as we have already noted, there is a range of sizes of motor units. A twitch of a large unit produces a much

greater contractile force than that of a small one. When a muscle is producing a small contraction, only the small units are used. As the contraction gets stronger, larger units are recruited, until all units are firing as fast as they can. As the contraction reduces, the units are decruited in reverse order, the large ones ceasing firing first. One benefit of this **orderly recruitment** is that contractions can be smoothly increased and decreased in strength.

A second and further sophistication is that there are various types of muscle fibre, for example:

- fatigue-resistant muscle fibres are able to remain active for long periods without tiring. Each fibre achieves this by having an aerobic metabolism, which means it needs a continuous supply of oxygen to keep working. This requires a good blood supply. This type of fibre produces relatively small amounts of contractile force and is typically found in a muscle's smaller motor units;

- fast-fatiguing muscle fibres are able to produce large contractile forces, but only for short periods. This type of fibre tires quickly because it relies on anaerobic metabolism (i.e. it works without oxygen). This can only be a short-term activity partly because if the by-products accumulated they would damage the muscle. It is typically found in a muscle's larger motor units.

The performance of these various fibre types underlies the everyday observation that it is not possible to maintain a very strong contraction in a muscle for very long.

All of the fibres in one motor unit are of the same type. The balance between different muscle fibre types found in a given muscle depends on that muscle's role.

◈   What type of fibre would you expect to find in power muscles, e.g. the muscles you use to lift a heavy box?

◆   Power muscles are used to produce large forces for a short time. They tend to have predominantly fast-fatiguing units.

◈   What type of fibre would you expect to find in muscles that are mostly used to maintain posture?

◆   Postural muscles must remain active for long periods in order to keep us upright, but they do not need to produce large contractile forces. They tend to have predominantly fatigue-resistant motor units.

These differences in the composition of muscles give rise to, for example, the different coloured meat in a roast chicken. The dark colour of the leg meat is due to the fact that the leg muscles (which are postural) contain mostly fatigue-resistant units whose extensive blood supply produces the colour. Conversely, the white meat of the wings is lighter in colour because the wing muscles (that in a chicken are only used occasionally and then only briefly) predominantly contain fast-fatiguing units.

Getting muscles to produce and then maintain just the right amount of contractile force is by no means easy. It is a job for a sophisticated control system. We know that this control system is in the CNS, but exactly where in the CNS is it? Interestingly, it is thought that most of the neural circuitry underlying asynchronous firing and orderly recruitment is in the spinal cord, in and around the alpha motor neurons. When we make a voluntary movement such as lifting a cup of tea to our lips, signals descend from the brain to the spinal cord 'asking' certain muscle groups

to contract. (We return to this later in the chapter.) But the brain does not need to concern itself with the details of how the muscle contraction will be produced, which motor units to use, how many to use, or how fast they should fire. It just asks for a certain level of contraction and the spinal cord 'works out' how to produce it.

This sort of division of labour is widespread within our movement control systems. As you begin to realize just how complex a task these systems carry out, you will understand why breaking the job down into smaller pieces in this way makes sense. But it makes the study of these systems harder because we cannot usually find any one part of the CNS that is controlling a given movement or posture. There are always many parts working together, each doing their own bit, and each 'talking' to the other parts involved.

2.7.4   The length–tension relationship in a muscle

The length of a muscle is not constant. Its length at any one moment depends on the position (i.e. angle) of the joint it crosses. The contractile force that a muscle can produce depends on the length at which it is working. This is the **length– tension relationship**.

One very important consequence of this length–tension relationship for our movement control is that a given neural input (or drive) to a muscle does not produce a given force output. What you get out of a muscle depends not only on how hard you drive it but also on its length at the time. From this we can predict that, in order to control our movement adequately, the CNS must have some way of sensing from moment to moment the length of all of the muscles in our body. You will see in the next section that it does indeed have access to this large amount of ever-changing information, and that if, through disease, it loses this facility, its ability to control movement is hugely impaired.

Summary of Section 2.7

Skeletal muscles span joints and can move the joints when they contract. Muscles cannot actively lengthen so they need to work in antagonistic pairs to move joints. Antagonistic pairs can also stiffen a joint by both contracting at the same time. This is known as co-contraction. In some cases this will result in there being no movement, in which case it is an isometric contraction – the muscles develop tension but do not shorten.

The muscle cell is called a muscle fibre and, like a neuron, it is an excitable cell that develops action potentials.

The smallest possible unit of motor activity is a brief contraction (called a twitch) occurring in a single motor unit, which comprises one alpha motor neuron and the muscle fibres that it innervates. A sustained and steady level of muscle contraction requires the asynchronous firing of many motor units. A stronger contraction is obtained by recruiting more motor units and/or by increasing the firing frequency of active motor units.

Motor units vary in size and in how rapidly they fatigue. The force output is dependent on the length of the muscle at the moment that the motor unit is activated. Thus to control movement the CNS must have a considerable amount of detailed information about the relative position of the various parts of the body.

Activity 2.2

You can demonstrate that your CNS 'knows' about your muscles' length–tension relationships in the following way.

1 Grasp the first two fingers of your left hand with all of the fingers of your right hand (Figure 2.16).

2 Squeeze the fingers on your left hand as hard as you can without hurting them. What position is your right wrist in? You should find that it is straight.

3 Try first extending and then flexing your right wrist (about 45°) and in each position try squeezing the fingers on your left hand. You should find that the strength of the squeeze is considerably reduced in these two positions.

A *power grip* like this is produced not by the muscles of the hand but by those of the forearm, in the tendons running across the wrist into the hand. You can convince yourself of this by looking at your forearm whilst making and releasing such a grip. You will see the forearm moving as the muscles contract and then relax. As you flex and extend the wrist, you change the length at which these muscles are working. They are set up to be at optimal working length when the wrist is straight. When you flex and extend the wrist the relevant muscles are respectively shorter and longer than optimal and therefore cannot produce so much force output. What is interesting is that, without knowing any of this, you probably started off with your wrist straight. This is because, where possible, your CNS uses your muscles at their optimal working length, especially where large force output is required.

Incidentally, the good guys in gangster films know all about length–tension relationships. The good guy forcibly flexes the bad guy's wrist to get the bad guy to release his grip on the gun. The gun obligingly drops to the floor. It really does work – but this is not one to try at home!

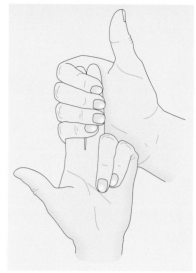

Figure 2.16   Grasping the first two fingers of the left hand with the right hand in a *power grip*.

2.8   Sensory input to the motor system

At the beginning of the chapter we quoted Charles Sherrington's observation that all paths in the brain led (directly or indirectly) to motor output. We can add that all paths into the brain come from sensory input. We are very aware of the senses (or sensory modalities) that guide our actions in relation to the external environment: we cross the road when we see (and hear) that there are no approaching vehicles, we run to rescue the burning toast that we smell (and see smoking) and we spit out the vile tasting vinegar that our 'friend' put in a wine glass for a practical joke. By contrast, we are not consciously aware of the sensory input from our internal environment that tells us where our limbs are in space at any moment and what, if any, movement is taking place. This information is provided by our **proprioceptors**.

◆ Look at Figure 2.10a and identify the sensory receptor (i.e. the proprioceptor) involved in the muscle stretch reflex.

◆ The weight that is added to the hand causes the muscle to stretch. In turn, the **muscle spindle** triggers electrical activity at the tip of the sensory neuron, neuron 1, that innervates the stretched muscle. The sensory receptor shown in Figure 2.10a is the muscle spindle.

In fact, neuron 1 is a component of the muscle spindle (Figure 2.17). As you can see from the figure, the receptor consists of two different kinds of sensory neurons that are wrapped around a specialized group of muscle fibres known as *intrafusal*

fibres to distinguish them from the working skeletal muscle, which are *extrafusal* fibres. (Incidentally, the motor input to intrafusal fibres is provided by gamma motor neurons, as opposed to the alpha motor neurons that provide input to the extrafusal fibres.) The two kinds of afferent sensory neurons can be distinguished because they are different sizes. The larger fibres are called Ia fibres; the II fibres are thinner. The fibres entwine around different areas of the intrafusal fibres as shown in Figure 2.17b. The Ia fibres detect the initial stretching of the surrounding muscle, increasing the rate at which they fire action potentials as the stretch develops, but falling back to a steady rate of firing once the muscle maintains a particular length. By contrast, the group II fibres respond more slowly as the stretch develops and maintain their firing rate throughout the stretch (Figure 2.18).

◆   What is the name of the process whereby a receptor detects a physical stimulus and transforms it into a pattern of neural activity?

◆   The process is called transduction.

Mechanoreceptors, such as the muscle spindle, are stimulated by mechanical means. At the time of writing (2003) it is thought that the muscle stretch might literally pull open ion channels, but no one knows for certain how mechanical forces are transduced into neural signals by muscle spindles.

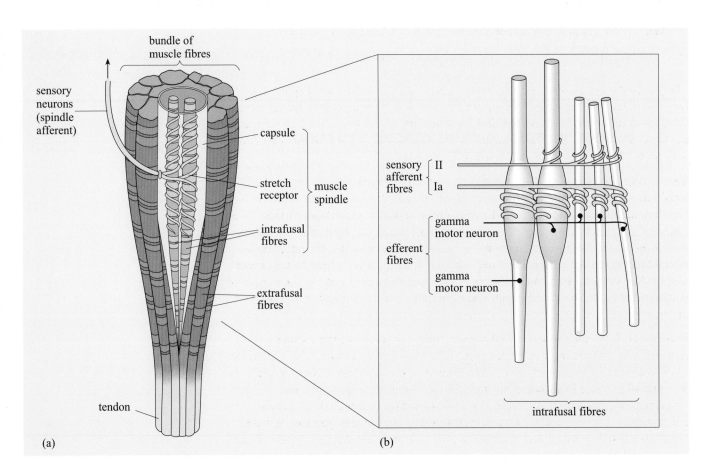

Figure 2.17   (a) Diagram of a muscle spindle showing how it lies encapsulated in skeletal muscle within a group of extrafusal muscle fibres. (b) Diagram showing the Ia afferent fibres with their free nerve endings wrapped around the central portions of the intrafusal muscle fibres and the II afferent fibres with their free endings wrapped around the extremities of the intrafusal fibres.

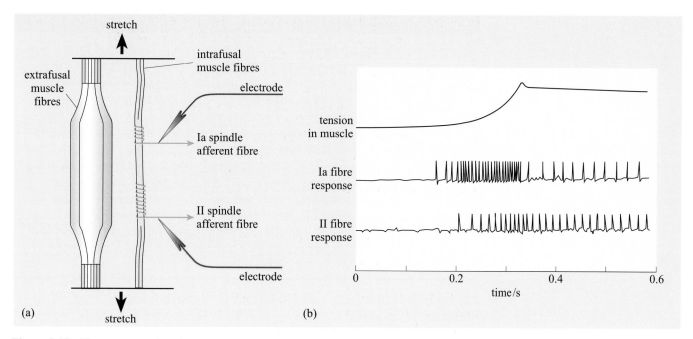

Figure 2.18   The responses given by muscle spindle afferent fibres when muscles are being passively stretched. (a) Diagram of the recording arrangement; (b) the traces obtained for muscle tension and firing patterns of the spindle afferent fibres.

◆   What is the name of the neural activity seen in a stimulated receptor?

◆   A stimulated receptor shows a receptor potential (Section 1.5.2).

Many receptor types, such as the photoreceptors in your eyes, can only generate a receptor potential. However, mechanoreceptors are modified sensory neurons and therefore have axonal membranes that can transmit action potentials. The receptor potential will trigger an action potential when the firing threshold for that particular neuron has been reached, as described in Chapter 1.

Thus the stretch on the muscle is transduced into a changed electrical potential within the muscle spindle sensory afferent fibres, the muscle spindles are excited and they increase the frequency with which they send action potentials to the CNS. These inform the CNS of the movement and/or of the new length of the muscle and therefore the new position of the joint. As we have already noted, this information is of central importance to our movement control systems. We will see in the course of this chapter that joint position information is used in many ways in the control of our movement. It also underlies our conscious sense of the position and movement of our bodies.

Information from the muscle spindles concerning the length of the muscles, together with signals from other receptors in the tendons and joints, give rise in the CNS to an internal representation of the relative positions of all the body parts. This is constantly updated and underlies the sense we have of the position and movement of our own bodies. This sense is called **proprioception**. Because we are never without proprioception (you cannot turn it off in the way you can turn off vision by closing your eyes), we tend not to be aware that we have it, but it is easy enough to demonstrate that we do.

Activity 2.3

Close your eyes and gently touch the tip of your nose with an index finger. Now ask yourself how you knew where the tip of your nose was. A perhaps more convincing demonstration requires an accomplice. With your left arm relaxed, get someone to flex and extend your left elbow back and forth in a random, unpredictable way. Get them sometimes to make fast movements, sometimes slow ones, sometimes small ones, sometime large ones, and to change direction unpredictably. With your right arm, match what they are doing to your left arm. You should find this quite easy. You will probably notice there is only a short lag between the left and right arms. Now close your eyes and do the same thing again. Your friend will almost certainly tell you that you are just as good (or better!) at matching or *tracking* your left arm movements with your eyes closed as you were with your eyes open. You are following the imposed movements of your left arm using your proprioceptors which, as we have said, include the muscle spindles.

One thing that this activity demonstrates is that the information from our proprioceptors is available to consciousness. However, it turns out that only a subset of the information is made available, and then in a highly processed form. (Can you see parallels here with the visual system described in Book 1, Chapter 4?) For example, we know where our various body segments (e.g. head, forearm) are with respect to one another and even where the various parts (e.g. nose) of each segment are on that segment. But we have no conscious knowledge of how long our muscles are or of how much we are contracting them. This information is available to the CNS but it just does not reach consciousness. It is however used in some form by our movement control systems. When, through disease, the CNS loses access to information from the muscle and joint receptors, a person is initially completely unable to move or even sit up in bed. This is perhaps surprising. One way of understanding why it might be so is to use an analogy. If you are trying to find your way somewhere using a map, it is not sufficient simply to know where you are going, you also need to know where you are otherwise you cannot work out in which direction to go. Similarly for the CNS, in order to move a body part it needs to know where it is now, otherwise the CNS cannot even work out which muscles to use to get it to where you want it to go. Since it is the information from proprioceptors which tells the CNS where the body parts are, losing this information renders it incapable of moving the body, or even of holding it in a desired posture. With time, people suffering this loss are able to regain some ability to move by using their vision. However, their movement control is hugely impoverished to the point that they are generally unable ever again to live independently.

The total loss of proprioceptive input is, mercifully, a rare complaint. The sensory input from the muscle spindle (represented by neuron 1 in Figure 2.10a) will normally enter the CNS and become available to the motor control system. We will quickly revise the route the information takes. On entering the spinal cord via a dorsal root, a spindle afferent divides, sending branches up and down to other levels of the cord, and also up to the brain. Another branch of the spindle afferent enters the grey matter at that level (segment) where it further divides extensively. These branches synapse directly with the alpha motor neurons of the muscle from which the afferent fibre originates. Through this branching, the fibre will synapse with all of the muscle's motor neurons.

◆   How many connections will this involve?

◆   For a large muscle this could be as many as 1000; even for a small muscle there will be at least 100 motor units.

When you bear in mind that a large muscle could have as many as 500 muscle spindles, each synapsing with about 1000 motor neurons, you start to realize that the 'wiring diagram' is going to look a bit scary (500 000 connections). So traditionally the situation is simplified, for example in Figure 2.10a just one spindle afferent synapsing onto one motor neuron is shown. This extensive connectivity between the stretch receptors in a muscle and its motor innervation gives rise to the stretch reflex that has already been described in Book 1, Section 3.3.2 in relation to placing a weight onto your hand. A much quoted example of a stretch reflex is the tendon jerk, so called because hitting a tendon causes a jerk in the limb. Tendon jerks are routinely used by physicians, particularly neurologists, to test the integrity of the afferent pathways and the conditions in the spinal cord. Your GP may have 'tested your reflexes' in this way by tapping your patellar tendon with a tendon hammer (the knee jerk). Indeed, a reflex pathway as direct as this is virtually impossible to switch off just with an act of will. However, you will see later in this chapter that other more complex reflex pathways are very much under your conscious control.

2.9   Coordination of muscle action about a joint

We noted from Figure 2.12 that an antagonist pair, e.g. biceps and triceps, have to work together to produce movement of the elbow joint. In order for the joint to flex, biceps must contract but triceps must relax, and vice versa. The spindle afferents from a muscle make connections with the motor neurons of that muscle (i.e. the homonymous muscle) and also with those of the muscle's antagonist. However, whereas the effect on the muscle's own motor neurons is excitatory, that on the antagonist's neurons is inhibitory.

◆   How does an excitatory input from the muscle spindle afferents bring about an inhibitory response in the antagonist's neurons?

◆   The pathway includes a short interneuron (a neuron which does not leave the spinal cord) that forms an inhibitory synapse with the antagonist motor neuron (Figure 2.10). This connectivity is known as reciprocal innervation (Book 1, Section 3.3.2).

The effect is that a stretch of biceps not only produces a reflex contraction in biceps, but also a reflex relaxation in triceps. This sort of arrangement is extended for more complex joints like the shoulder and hip that can move in various ways and have a number of pairs of antagonistic muscles crossing them.

These observations suggest that the 'wiring' together in the spinal cord of the neurons that control muscles crossing a joint has the purpose of opposing external movement, or perturbation, of that joint. In other words, muscle stretch reflexes do not exist to oppose stretch of muscles per se, but to oppose perturbations to joints.

◆   Can you think of any circumstances when we might need a motor system that could rapidly adjust to external forces?

◆   A slightly dramatic answer would be that we need such a system to avoid being blown over by a strong gust of wind whilst waving to granny! You might also have thought of the slippery rocks scenario, mentioned at the beginning of this chapter.

We considered earlier that, for a large muscle, some 500 spindle afferent fibres might each branch some 1000 times in order to synapse on all of the muscle's motor neurons, producing a complex pattern of connections within the spinal cord. But just reflect for a moment on the 'wiring' implications of what we've just been discussing. We have not yet considered the input to each motor neuron.

◆   To what extent do synaptic inputs converge onto a motor neuron?

◆   It is thought that each motor neuron receives somewhere in the region of 10 000 separate synaptic inputs.

The congestion is beyond imagination. What can be the advantages of this hugely elaborate system? Would a simpler system suffice? Unfortunately, at this point we hit our first brick wall. Nobody really knows the answer to these seemingly simple questions. You can at least console yourself with the thought that, already, we've just about reached the *cutting edge* (Book 3, Section 2.2.1).

One part of the answer seems to be that this elaborate system helps in the control of voluntary (i.e. willed) movements. Imagine that you are lifting a large bowl of water up onto a shelf in front of you. The water in the bowl moves around as you lift it. As it slops away from you it assists your lifting movement, as it slops towards you it impedes it. This will stretch respectively biceps and triceps whose stretch reflexes will help to reduce the instability caused by the movement of the water. It is also thought that our own muscles cause similar small instabilities during movement that the spinal stretch reflex helps to 'iron out' (less dramatic than the gust of wind, but just as important).

Another part of the answer is nothing to do with reflexes at all. For, as first mentioned in Book 1, Section 3.3.2, it seems that the brain uses these spinal circuits in the actual production of voluntary movement. As we have already noted, voluntary movements arise through signals descending from the brain to the spinal cord. Descending fibres typically branch extensively in the spinal cord. Some synapse both with a muscle's alpha motor neurons and with the interneurons we have already met that inhibit its antagonist. Thus signals descending in these fibres both activate a muscle and relax its antagonist. The brain does not have to do each of these things separately. In fact, the descending signal could be thought of as specifying, or coding, a movement of a joint rather than muscle activity, the spinal cord translating this instruction into the muscle actions required. This is another example of a job being split into components with different parts of the CNS each contributing their bit.

We have already noted that sometimes what is required is not movement at a joint, but resistance to movement (remember the writing a letter and electric sander examples). We stiffen a joint by contracting both muscles of an antagonist pair together (co-contracting). This raises a problem. It's a bit tricky so worth taking slowly. If you contract biceps, this will stretch triceps causing a stretch reflex which will activate triceps (which is okay because you want co-contraction) and inhibit biceps (which is *not* okay, because you want co-contraction), and vice versa. Have another look at Figure 2.10. It would seem that the spinal circuitry coordinates the muscles crossing a joint for movement of that joint, not for stiffening it. So how do we co-contract? The answer is that the brain can change the way the spinal circuits work. Using descending fibres that have a strong inhibitory influence on the interneurons we have been discussing, the brain can effectively turn reciprocal innervation off. This brain mechanism allows the spinal circuitry to stiffen a joint effectively.

It may be that much of the elaborate connectivity in the spinal cord exists to provide elementary patterns of coordination of the muscles crossing a joint, which the brain can use and switch between. The spinal cord takes care of some of the detail leaving the brain free to deal with the wider picture. There is however a caveat here. Although something along these lines seems to be going on, the evidence for it all is still rather sketchy. We are a long way from understanding all that is going on in these complex spinal circuits, and they are still very much a focus of current research.

Summary of Sections 2.8 and 2.9

Sensory input from joints and muscles, which tells the CNS where the limbs are, is provided by proprioceptors such as the muscle spindles that detect muscle stretch. It is proprioception that underlies our conscious sense of the position and movement of our bodies. Not all proprioceptive information is available to consciousness, for example we are not aware of the lengths of muscles. In the absence of proprioception our ability to move is hugely impaired.

Normally, proprioceptive input drives the stretch reflex and in addition the sensory afferent fibre makes connections in other segments of the spinal cord as well as feeding into ascending pathways to the brain.

The connections just within one segment of the spinal cord are awesome. A muscle might have 500 muscle spindles, each synapsing with around 1000 motor neurons. Each of these motor neurons could have around 10 000 other inputs. However, when we draw diagrams of the stretch reflex we simplify this to show one sensory afferent synapsing with one motor neuron.

The role of this complex circuitry is uncertain, but it may be that spinal circuits code for different tasks (e.g. opposing perturbations about a joint, flexing joints, stabilizing joints by co-contracting muscles), and that the brain selects which circuit needs to dominate at any one time.

2.10   Experimental investigation of muscle reflexes

So far we have stated that muscles exhibit stretch reflexes, but we have not looked at the response in any detail. In this section we will do just that and uncover some hitherto unexpected sophistication.

One way of studying the response of muscles to stretch would be to measure the contractile force produced. But in most circumstances it is easier to measure the electrical activity – the action potentials that give rise to the contraction. This technique is called electromyography (Box 2.1).

Box 2.1   Electromyography

We have already seen that a muscle produces contractile force when action potentials occur in its fibres. In certain circumstances, these action potentials can be recorded intracellularly using a microelectrode, just as we might in a neuron (Book 3, Section 2.4.1). However, since it is usual for a large number of muscle fibres to be firing at the same time, which produces a considerable electrical disturbance in and around the muscle, we can usually pick up the electrical activity very simply with electrodes on the surface of the skin. This technique is known as surface electromyography (surface EMG).

Figure 2.19 shows the kind of result obtained when we use surface EMG to observe the response to a tendon tap. The recording apparatus is triggered by a micro-switch in the tendon hammer so that the trace begins at the instant the tendon is struck.

It is easy to misinterpret this type of record by confusing it with an intracellular measurement. Bear in mind that here we are not looking at one action potential from inside one muscle fibre or one neuron, but at the combined effect of action potentials in hundreds or thousands of muscle fibres – a *compound action potential*, as seen from outside the cells producing them.

Electromyography is widely used both in research and in the clinic as an aid to diagnosis of early stages of muscle or nerve dysfunction, for example muscular sclerosis and motor neuron disease.

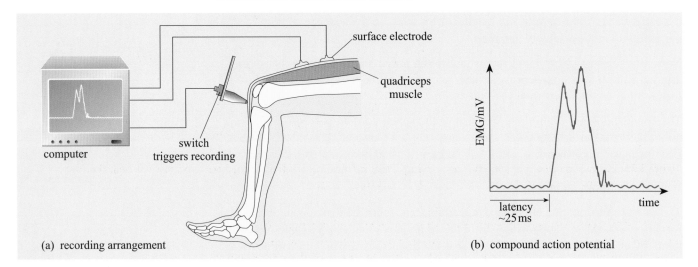

(a) recording arrangement

(b) compound action potential

Figure 2.19   (a) Experimental arrangement for recording a tendon jerk in the quadriceps muscle. Electrodes stuck to the skin over the muscle pick up the electrical disturbance that occurs when the muscle's fibres twitch. The tendon hammer is instrumented such that the recording apparatus is triggered at the instant the tendon is struck. (b) A typical tendon jerk trace. Since the trace was started at the moment the tendon was struck, the time between the start of the trace and the beginning of the response is a measure of the latency of the reflex.

From a trace such as that in Figure 2.19 the time between the stimulus (tendon tap) and the response (muscle activity) can be deduced. The time interval between the stimulus that evokes a reflex and the consequent response is called the latency of the reflex. In this case it is about 25 ms. This is the time taken for the tap to stretch the muscle, the stretch to excite the muscle spindles, the action potentials in the spindle afferents to travel to the spinal cord, the signal to cross the single synapse and excite the motor neurons, the action potentials to travel in the efferent fibres to the muscle, and the signal to cross the neuromuscular junctions and instigate action potentials in the muscle fibres. So there is quite a lot happening in the one-fortieth of a second that it takes this reflex response to occur. Reflexes are quick!

2.10.1   Long-latency stretch responses

Tapping a muscle's tendon causes a very brief and small stretch. When a muscle is subjected to a slower stretch, more like those that occur in the course of normal movement, its response can be more complex. Figure 2.20 shows the responses of two muscles, flexor pollicis longus (FPL: the thumb flexor muscle) and biceps, to slower stretches. In this experiment the muscles were stretched by a motor that pulled on the thumb (FPL) or the forearm (biceps) (Figure 2.20a). In one experimental condition the participants made no attempt to resist the pull of the motor. In another, they were instructed to pull against the motor as soon as they felt it begin to pull them.

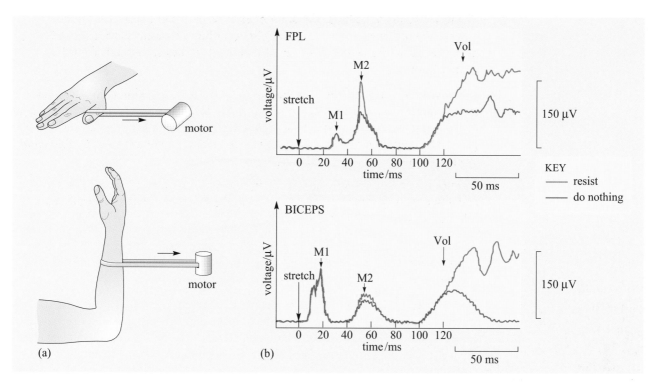

Figure 2.20   (a) Experimental arrangements for stretching a thumb flexor muscle (FPL) and the biceps muscle. (b) Typical traces obtained. These have three phases labelled M1, M2 and Vol. See text for explanation.

The resulting traces are very different from those obtained with a tendon jerk. We now have a complex response with three separate phases. The first, called M1, occurs in the biceps at between 15 ms and 20 ms after the onset of the stretch and is due to the spinal circuit that we have been discussing.

◆   Why is the latency of this response shorter than that in the quadriceps muscle (see Figure 2.19b)?

◆   The response occurs more rapidly because the biceps is closer to the spinal cord and therefore the afferent and efferent fibres are shorter. Although peripheral nerves conduct (propagate) action potentials fairly quickly (the fastest fibres in humans conduct at about $50\,\mathrm{m\,s^{-1}}$), the conduction delay involved is still significant and gives rise to different reflex latencies in different muscles.

Thus the latency of the M1 response in FPL is longer than in biceps (and about the same as that in quadriceps).

The second phase of the response, M2, occurs about 50 ms after the onset of the stretch. This phase represents another component of the stretch reflex. It has a longer latency because it travels further through the CNS. We'll come back to M2 in a moment. The third phase of the response, labelled Vol, is the voluntary part of the response. We will be discussing voluntary movement in the next chapter, but these results give us an opportunity to begin to think about it now. It is clear that when the participants in the experiment intended to resist the pull of the motor there was a much larger contraction in the muscle, but this was not evident until some 120 ms after the stimulus for both muscles. No matter how hard the participants might have

tried to make this component of the response faster, they would not have been able to do so.

◆ Why do you think this delay cannot be decreased?

◆ Although the distance now includes a trip to and from the brain, this extra distance is only a small part of the story. In this neural circuit there is going to be considerably more processing occurring in the brain – and more neurons involved means more synaptic delay.

The thing about a voluntary response, which distinguishes it from a reflex response, is that it can take any form you like. Instead of asking the participants to pull back against the motor when they felt it pull on them, the experimenters could have asked them to shout 'now!', raise the other arm, or tap a foot. But whatever form the voluntary response took, it would not have occurred more quickly than about 120 ms after the stimulus. So although voluntary responses are much more flexible than reflex responses, they are nowhere near as fast.

The fact that reflex responses can occur at such short latency suggests that part of their role in movement control might be to make adjustments as quickly as possible (more about this later). It used to be assumed that their disadvantage was that they are inflexible, the same input (stimulus) always producing the same output (response).

◆ Look at Figure 2.20b. Does the same stimulus (a slow stretch) always produce a response of the same magnitude?

◆ The M1 responses for both muscles are the same regardless of the participant's intention. However particularly noticeable in the case of FPL, the M2 response is not quite the same in the two experimental conditions. It seems to be larger when the participant was attempting to resist the motor's pull.

The M2 deflection does not represent a voluntary response. The participant could not have said 'now!' or tapped a foot at this latency. The M2 response is not flexible to anywhere near this degree, but it seems that neither is it inflexible in the way that the M1 response is. The M2 response seems to be something in-between a reflex and voluntary response.

Responses like M2 are known as **long-latency stretch responses** and they are very interesting indeed. For not only can they change in size according to the participant's intention, but they can also appear in muscles other than the one stretched, according to the circumstances. For example if in the experiment depicted in Figure 2.20 the participant is standing up, the pull on the forearm will tend to disturb their balance, pulling them over forwards. Under these conditions we see responses in the calf muscles at about the same latency as the M2 in biceps at approximately 50 ms (Figure 2.21). When balance is disturbed in this way the body will begin to fall forwards. This will stretch the calf muscles and thus evoke a stretch reflex. So finding a stretch response in the calf muscles seems to make sense. But when we measure the position and movement of the participant's knees during the experiment we find that the knees move forwards (and therefore the calf muscles are stretched) *after*, not before, the response in the calf muscles (Figure 2.21b). Obviously, a response cannot occur before the stimulus that evokes it, so we have to conclude that movement of the ankle joints and consequent stretch of the calf muscles is *not* the stimulus.

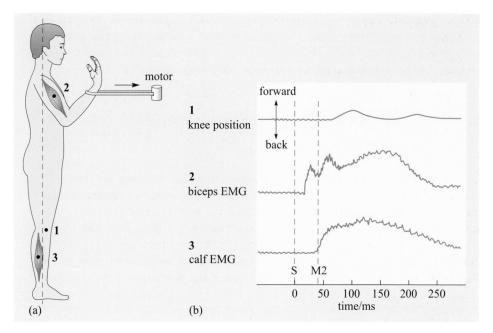

Figure 2.21   A standing subject's biceps muscle is stretched by a forwards pull to the forearm at time 'S' (the stimulus) sufficient in strength to pull the whole body forwards, partly by moving the ankle joint. Long-latency stretch responses (M2) are seen in the calf muscles, but these occur before the ankle joint position (as measured by knee position) changes, and therefore before the calf muscles are stretched. Further experiments confirm that the responses in the calf muscles are due to stretch of biceps. This is an example of the 'gating' of long-latency stretch responses into distant muscle groups that presumably occurs to reduce the disturbance to balance caused by a predictable stimulus.

It turns out that the stimulus is the stretch of biceps. As soon as you stand up, the CNS 'realizes' that now the pull to the forearm is going to pull the whole body forwards, and so, in preparation, it makes a connection that routes signals from biceps' stretch receptors down to the calf muscles. As a result, an M2-type response appears in the calf muscles following stretch of biceps by the motor. The advantage of this strategy for the CNS is that it gets a useful, or functional, response in the calf muscles at 50 ms latency. A voluntary response will also appear in the calf muscles but, of course, this will not even begin until at least 120 ms after the stimulus. In a situation where the body is rapidly moving towards instability, speed is of the essence. The longer the CNS leaves it to respond, the more precarious the situation becomes and the more difficult it is to make a correction. The CNS uses all available information in presetting its reflex circuits. For example, if a support is placed against the participant's chest such that they can no longer be pulled forwards, responses are no longer found in the calf. If the stimulus could be either a pull or a push, and the CNS has no way of knowing in advance which it is to be, again responses are not found in the calf.

So, although some reflexes such as the muscle stretch reflex are relatively stereotyped and inflexible, others, like these long-latency responses, are enormously adaptable. It is interesting to note that what the CNS is doing here is making a best guess or prediction about what is going to happen in the future and preparing its reflex circuits accordingly. You will see in the following chapter that predictions of this sort are a very important aspect of motor control.

In fact, predictions are a very important aspect of life in general. Being good at predicting not only what is going to happen to you, but also what other people are going to do, based on whatever limited information happens to be available at the present, confers significant advantage on an individual. Might the way we use our nervous systems for predicting the future be based on how we use them for predicting how our bodies are going to move? If, as we suggested in the introduction to this chapter, nervous systems originally evolved to control movement, and only later started to be used for all of the complex business of social living, this might well be the case. Food for thought?

Getting back to long-latency stretch responses, there has been a great deal of debate about where in the CNS all of this switching of stretch responses from one muscle to another actually occurs. Once again we have reached the cutting edge and there are no simple answers. It does seem however that at least part of the job is done by the motor cortex. We have already had some discussion of the role of the primary motor cortex in Book 1, Section 3.4.6. We noted that it plays a dominant role in motor control and is involved in the execution of our most finely graded and conscious actions, for example the precise manipulation of objects with the hands such as playing the piano. The fact that there is also involvement of the motor cortex in these stretch responses suggests that their control is something of a priority for the motor systems.

Some of the most convincing evidence that long-latency stretch responses are routed via the cortex, (the **trans-cortical hypothesis**), has come from observations of individuals with Klippel–Feil syndrome. This is a condition in which there is a congenital abnormality in the upper cervical spine (the upper-neck region), the part of the spinal cord in which the alpha motor neurons that innervate the arm and hand muscles are located. Normally, axons descending from the brain's motor cortex that control hand muscles synapse with motor neurons innervating the hand on just one side of the body (the left hemisphere controls the right side of the body, and vice versa). In Klippel–Feil syndrome, however, the cortical axons are thought to branch in the cervical cord, synapsing with motor neurons innervating both hands (Figure 2.22a). The connections remain specific such that a given cortical neuron controls the same, or homologous, muscle in each hand. As a result, people with this syndrome suffer from mirror movements of the hands.

Figure 2.22 (a) In Klippel–Feil syndrome cortical axons are thought to branch in the cervical cord, synapsing with motor neurons innervating homologous muscles in the two hands. Note: motor neuron is green; sensory neuron is black. (b) In a Klippel–Feil individual, stretch of a muscle in one hand produces a long-latency stretch response in both that muscle and the homologous muscle in the other hand. This is good evidence that long-latency responses can be mediated via a trans-cortical pathway.

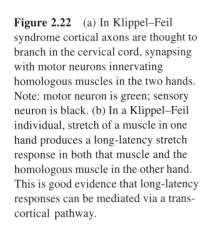

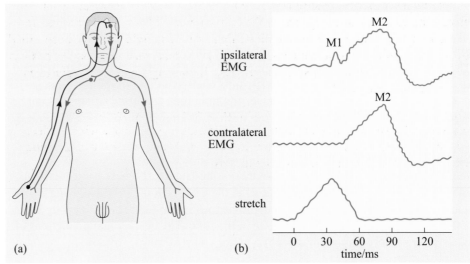

When they make an intentional movement of one hand, the other hand involuntarily does the same thing.

In an individual with Klippel–Feil syndrome, stretching a muscle in the hand on one side produces a large M2 response not only in that muscle, but also in the homologous muscle in the other hand (Figure 2.22b). This of course does not happen in normal individuals and is good evidence for the existence of a trans-cortical stretch-reflex pathway. This is a very good example of the way in which a neurological abnormality or disease can help us understand the way in which the normal or healthy nervous system works.

Summary of Section 2.10

When a muscle is slowly stretched the surface EMG displays three phases: M1 is the rapid monosynaptic stretch reflex with a latency of about 25 ms; Vol is the voluntary response (e.g. resisting the contraction) and has a latency of 120 ms; M2 is the long-latency stretch reflex and occurs about 50 ms after the stimulus. M2 is larger if the stimulus can be anticipated, as when the individual has been told to resist a predictable stimulus (i.e. to pull against the motor that stretches the muscle). But, intriguingly, M2 is also sometimes found in muscles other than the one being stretched. We have deduced from experiments that M2 is a predictive response that can be given in some circumstances, for example to oppose the tendency to topple forwards if grabbed by the arms.

The trans-cortical hypothesis states that M2 responses are routed via the motor cortex, based on evidence from individuals with Klippel–Feil syndrome. These people have cortical axons that branch in the cervical cord and synapse with motor neurons, innervating both hands (normally one hand only would be innervated). A stretch to one hand generates M2 activity in both that muscle and the homologous muscle in the other hand.

2.11   Summary of Chapter 2

In this chapter we have seen how visual information might be processed to enable us to recognize our grandmother and how proprioception is needed to allow us to move our muscles appropriately as we wave to her. Even simple movements such as waving must involve precise and complex orchestration of neuronal signals to ensure the coordinated movement of the huge numbers of muscle fibres that are needed for this activity. These complicated patterns of muscle activity are specified by neural circuits in the spinal cord, but there is evidence that the motor cortex can be involved, without our conscious awareness, in making anticipatory adjustments to the circuits being used.

Thus far we have only investigated the neural circuits responsible for reflex reactions. Whilst reflexes may assist us in maintaining our balance when jostled, waving is clearly not a reflex response. In the next chapter we will examine how we control voluntary movements such as waving.

Learning outcomes for Chapter 2

After studying this chapter, you should be able to:

2.1 Recognize definitions and applications of each of the terms printed in **bold** in the text.

2.2 Demonstrate an understanding of the ways in which the characteristics of the visual field are coded and conveyed to the brain.

2.3 Explain how the study of individuals with brain damage, together with the use of brain-imaging techniques, has helped in the elucidation of the neural pathways involved in visual processing and motor control.

2.4 Describe the properties of skeletal muscle and the ways in which it is activated by alpha motor neurons.

2.5 Describe how muscle spindles can serve as stretch detectors and explain why not all proprioceptive information is available to consciousness.

2.6 Demonstrate an awareness of the complexity of spinal circuits.

2.7 Give evidence for believing that the motor cortex can be involved in some reflex responses.

Questions for Chapter 2

Question 2.1   (Learning outcome 2.2)

Students emerging from a lecture on face recognition are overheard saying that they still do not understand how light reaches the brain. What would you say to them to help their understanding?

Question 2.2   (Learning outcome 2.3)

Evidence that the fusiform face area (FFA) is specialized for face recognition is ambiguous. In this chapter we have suggested that the contradictory evidence might demonstrate that the FFA exhibits neural plasticity. What other factor might account for the contradictory nature of the evidence?

Question 2.3   (Learning outcome 2.4)

What type of muscle fibres would you expect to find predominately in the wing muscles of migratory birds? How could they maximize output from these muscles?

Question 2.4   (Learning outcome 2.5)

Which of the following statement(s) are appropriate descriptions of the muscle spindle?

A   The muscle spindle lies in parallel with the working muscle.

B   The muscle spindle contracts to exert the force that moves joints in protective reflexes.

C   The muscle spindle monitors the extent/degree of stretch of working muscle.

D   The muscle spindle activates the distal region of an associated sensory neuron.

Question 2.5   (Learning outcomes 2.3, 2.6 and 2.7)

What is the relevance of Klipper–Feil syndrome to the trans-cortical hypothesis?

THE CONTROL OF MOVEMENT

3.1 Introduction

In Book 1, Section 4.5.1, we confronted some of the difficulties in studying the initiation of deliberate movements when we looked into Libet's experiments on freedom of action (i.e. free will). So it may seem strange that in a course that has the brain as its primary focus, we did not start our detailed investigations of movement control by studying the brain, preferring instead to move to the other end of the CNS to explore the relationships between the alpha motor neurons and the muscle fibres that they innervate. In fact, we started there because this is where we have the most understanding; the systems you have just studied in Chapter 2 were relatively simple. By contrast, integrating sensory information with past experience, in order to inform decision making so that we select appropriate actions, is complex as well as being poorly understood. We do not have space to explore it fully here.

Instead, let us return to the street where we first encountered granny so that we can review once more the problems with which the CNS must grapple. When you *see* your granny, a number of sensory circuits are activated, including the major cortical pathways, the dorsal and ventral streams, and non-cortical pathways such as the projection to the superior colliculi. These pathways are processing different aspects of the sensory information in parallel (see Section 1.6.2). The cortical pathways initially project to unimodal association areas in the occipital and temporal lobes, but from there they project to multimodal association areas such as the posterior parietal cortex, the temporal association cortex, the parahippocampal cortex and the cingulate cortex (as discussed in Book 1, Section 3.4.6). The activity in these areas enables you to link your total sensory experience with emotion, memory and learning.

You recognize granny and, knowing that she is hard of hearing, you do not call to her. Instead you wave. To allow this to happen, sensory information must be available to the area where motor activity is planned. This seems to be the frontal lobes. The prefrontal association areas also receive input from the thalamus and the limbic system (amygdala and cingulate cortex). Thus memory and emotion are again linked, this time to the planning process. Patients with damage to frontal lobes, such as Phineas Gage (Book 1, Section 1.1.4), have difficulties using memory and/or experience to plan their actions. Their immediate responses may be inappropriate, and longer-term planning can be so disrupted that they become apathetic drifters, as Phineas Gage is reported to have done. On the other hand, if you see granny frequently, then you probably do not need to spend much time thinking about how you can attract her attention. Waving rather than hailing her may be an automatic response and, as with incoming sensory information, so with motor systems, there are many parallel pathways that can, directly or indirectly, drive the alpha motor neurons to move your arm. The motor cortex can be directly activated with minimal planning as we saw when studying the M2 long-latency response in Section 2.10.1. But the motor cortex has direct input from two other systems, the basal ganglia and the cerebellum, that make important contributions to the control of motor behaviour. These two systems influence the activity of the motor cortex in particular ways. The basal ganglia are especially implicated in the initiation of voluntary or willed movement such as waving. So we will look into their contribution first. Discussion of the cerebellum comes towards the end of this chapter.

Voluntary movement is any movement that you make of your own volition. It contrasts with reflex movement, which was originally conceived as an inevitable and stereotypical consequence of a given external stimulus. Although we have seen that reflexes can be much more flexible and adaptable than this, they are nothing like as flexible and adaptable as voluntary responses. Furthermore, voluntary movement does not require an external signal to initiate it. We often make movements that are entirely self-generated, such as in the example followed through in some detail in Book 1, Section 3.4.6, where we imagined an individual learning to play the piano using vision to guide finger movements. Waving at granny is also self-generated, in that waving is not an inevitable response to seeing granny any more than playing a chord is an inevitable response to seeing a piano.

◆   Although both movements cited above are internally generated, there is a fundamental difference in the way they are directed. What is this difference?

◆   The pianist's movements are guided precisely to an external stimulus: the keyboard. The chord is only played when the fingers make contact with the correct keys. The form waving takes is independent of an external cue, we choose how to move our arm about in space – we can make a large arm movement or a small one. We do not make a precise physical connection with an external stimulus.

It seems that the role of the basal ganglia may differ subtly in these two conditions. We will return to this point after a more general consideration of the evidence that the basal ganglia have a moderating effect on the control of movement.

3.2   The basal ganglia and movement control

In the 17th century the structures that we now call the basal ganglia (striatum and globus pallidus, the subthalamic nucleus and the substantia nigra) were known as the corpus striatum (the striped body). This relatively large structure of striped appearance holds a central position in the brain and is connected to other parts of the brain by a mass of prominent fibre tracts. It was therefore surmised that it was of central importance in coordinating incoming sensory information and initiating all motor activity. Over the next two centuries, as research interest turned to the cerebral cortex with its fascinatingly regular histology (see Figure 1.26a) and more was discovered about its importance to various mental activities, the corpus striatum was gradually stripped of its prominent role. But by the beginning of the 20th century it was becoming clear that it did have an important role in at least some motor activities because of the severe deficits that were seen in motor performance in disease states such as Parkinson's disease (Section 1.6.4).

In Section 1.6.4, we suggested that the basal ganglia's contribution to motor control might be in planning and motor strategy. Thus when we see granny a number of potential motor responses could be triggered but only one may be possible to execute. The basal ganglia are instrumental in determining which one is selected. Specifically, when you see your granny, which arm will you wave? Will you push your hair back from your eyes? Will you brush away the annoying fly that has settled on your nose? What will you do with the parcels you are carrying? But that is not all that the basal ganglia have to contend with. In Section 1.6.4 we said that patients with the basal ganglia disorder called Parkinson's disease lost the ability to make normal facial expressions. So we are reminded that we must think not only about which arm we

are going to wave but also about all the other motor activity such as the expression on our face (a smile of pleasure at this unexpected meeting), and our gait (we can run to greet her or put down our parcels and open our arms ready to give her a hug). From the many possibilities, the evidence is that it is within the basal ganglia that the 'decisions' are made. But on what information are the basal ganglia making these 'decisions'?

The major inputs to the basal ganglia are from the cortex and thalamus to the striatum (caudate nucleus and putamen). Of these, it is the cortex that makes the most substantial contribution with input from sensory, association and motor cortices. (In fact, the only regions of the cortex that do not provide *direct* input are the primary visual and the primary auditory cortices.) Furthermore, the different streams from the cortex to the basal ganglia are topographically mapped and remain distinct as they project from the basal ganglia to the output regions.

The outputs are back to the cortex (especially the frontal lobes) via the ventral anterior (VA) and ventrolateral (VL) nuclei of the thalamus, and to brainstem structures such as the superior colliculi as shown in Figure 3.1. (You may also find it useful to look at Figure 3.11 in Book 1.)

The basal ganglia sit at a kind of 'neural crossroads' and are in a good position to select motor output. (The term 'ganglia' is actually a misnomer; these structures are more correctly described as nuclei – see Book 1, Section 3.4.)

Figure 3.1 (a) Diagrammatic section through the forebrain and midbrain to show the relative locations of basal ganglia structures. (b) Diagrammatic representation of the major connections within the basal ganglia and between the basal ganglia and associated structures. Inhibitory cells and synapses are represented in red; excitatory cells are white. Endings that are both white and red indicate that the neurotransmitter released can have either an excitatory or inhibitory action on the presynaptic neuron.

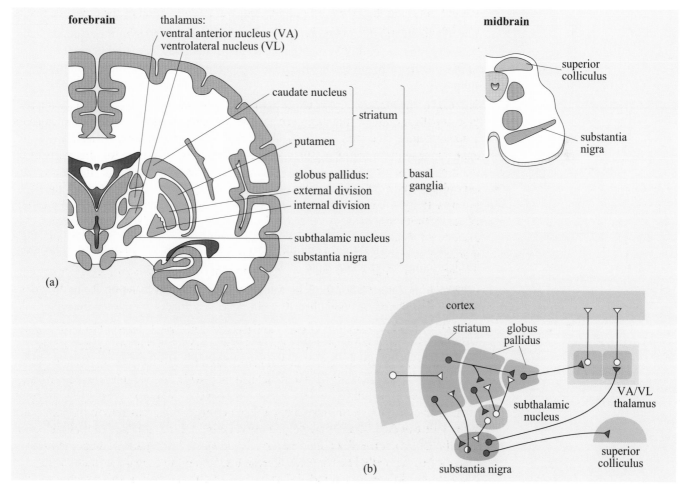

In section 1.6.4 we used the basal ganglia as an example of a neural network at work. We studied the interconnections between structures (nuclei) that together are termed the basal ganglia. We saw how different pathways can be traced through the basal ganglia based on the way that particular neurotransmitters are used. We also discussed two movement disorders, Parkinson's disease and Huntington's disease, which can be attributed to malfunctions of these pathways.

Evidence that the basal ganglia have a critical role in the selection of, and thereby the initiation of, movement comes from the experience of individuals with Parkinson's disease. Many of them find it hard to start to walk but once they get going they then find that it is not easy to stop. One activity that they find particularly difficult is pacing back and forth across a room.

◈   If these patients have a problem stopping, why do you think the basal ganglia are described as affecting initiation of motor activity?

◆   Control of muscle is a continuous activity. As you stop one activity another takes its place. Immediately you stop walking (which is a rhythmic activity) your muscles must contract differently to keep you upright and balanced (standing). Stopping and starting can be regarded as two sides of the same coin. So instead of saying that the basal ganglia initiate movement, we could have said that the basal ganglia select movements.

How do the basal ganglia control this switching between activities? Although we cannot give a precise answer to this question we can make a start by reflecting on how the basal ganglia and motor cortex are linked. Knowledge of these anatomical pathways and the ability to manipulate some of them has increased our understanding of the ways in which the basal ganglia are able to select motor output.

We first looked at these anatomical pathways in Book 1, Section 3.4.4. There we noted the direct input to the basal ganglia from the motor cortex. This gives the basal ganglia access to information about ongoing and planned motor activity. The loop is completed by an indirect pathway from basal ganglia to motor cortex.

◈   Which brain structure lies on the pathway from basal ganglia to motor cortex?

◆   The thalamus.

This means that the output from the basal ganglia has the potential to interrupt the flow of other information from thalamus to motor cortex.

Although the interrelationships between the structures that make up the basal ganglia are themselves complex, it is not necessary for us to concern ourselves with them here. What interests us is how the behavioural output in movement disorders such as Parkinson's disease and Huntington's disease can tell us something useful about the way that the neural output from the basal ganglia must function in normal, healthy individuals.

◈   From evidence of the movement disorder shown in Huntington's disease, what is the effect of the normal GABAergic output from the basal ganglia to the thalamus?

◆   GABA is an inhibitory neurotransmitter. Thus the normal GABAergic output from the basal ganglia has an inhibitory effect on the thalamic neurons to which it projects. In Huntington's disease this normal output is disrupted, i.e. the inhibitory 'brake' is removed. The effect is to 'allow' unwanted movements to occur. So the effect of the normal GABAergic output is to inhibit movement.

What is happening is that the basal ganglia are exerting their selection role by *preventing* movements from occurring most of the time. This is confirmed by recordings from the output neurons. These fire at very high frequencies (up to 100 per second) when behaviourally there is little or no physical activity. But when the basal ganglia output neurons stop firing this inhibition is removed, i.e. the thalamus can now send signals to the motor cortex that allows the motor cortex to initiate movement. (These output neurons from the motor cortex are called upper motor neurons, as distinct from the alpha motor neurons (lower motor neurons) that provide direct input to muscle fibres.) In these circumstances the basal ganglia are acting as a 'gate' controlling the thalamic output to the motor cortex (Figure 3.2).

Evidence that the basal ganglia permit the initiation of movement by a gating mechanism came from studies of eye movements. We have not considered eye movements at all so far, so we will introduce them here before returning to the subject in more detail when we consider the role of the cerebellum.

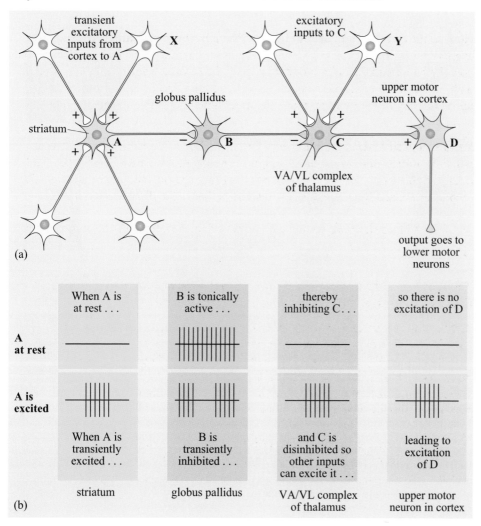

Figure 3.2   A chain of neurons arranged in a disinhibitory circuit. (a) Diagram of the connections between two inhibitory neurons A and B and an excitatory neuron C. (b) Pattern of the action potential activity of cells A, B and C when A is at rest, and when neuron A fires transiently as a result of its excitatory inputs. Such circuits are central to gating operations of the basal ganglia. X and Y are excitatory inputs to the inhibitory circuit.

There are only twelve muscles controlling our two eyes (i.e. six per eye) so the oculomotor system is the simplest of the motor control systems to study. There are six subsystems. One initiates rapid orienting eye movements called *saccades*. These provide a fixation system that keeps the fovea focused on a place of interest (Book 1, Section 4.5.3). The link from basal ganglia to the motor neurons controlling eye movement is not via the thalamus but via the superior colliculi. It has been observed that neurons in the superior colliculi fire prior to the initiation of a saccade. At other times there is a background rate of firing from the basal ganglia cells that project to the superior colliculi (i.e. these cells are tonically active), and the cells from the superior colliculi to the eye muscles are quiescent. Only when the tonic activity from the basal ganglia ceases do these superior colliculi neurons fire (Figure 3.3). In other words the normal output from the basal ganglia is to keep the 'gate' closed.

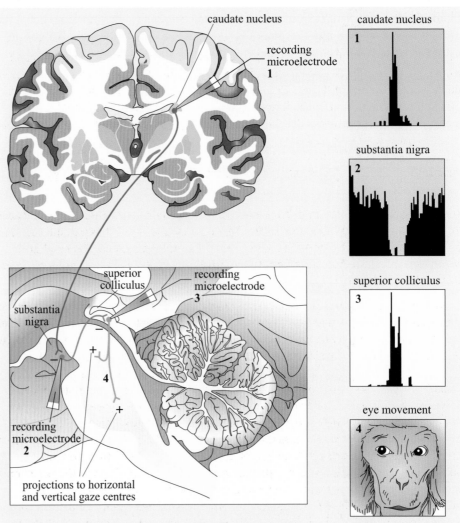

Figure 3.3   The role of basal ganglia disinhibition in the generation of saccadic eye movements. 1 An excitatory input from the cerebral cortex causes cells in the caudate nucleus (which is part of the striatum) to fire briefly. 2 Cells in the substantia nigra have been tonically active but the consequence of the burst of activity in the caudate nucleus is to interrupt this activity, i.e. they are inhibited for a brief spell. 3 The result of their momentarily ceasing to fire is that the upper motor neurons of the superior colliculus are no longer inhibited ('gate' opened). They can generate a burst of action potentials that command a saccade (4).

Another approach to understanding the basal ganglia's role in movement control has been to inject GABA agonists into the output nuclei.

◆   What does an agonist do?

◆   Agonists mimic the activity of the neurotransmitter (see Section 1.4.4).

This treatment temporarily interrupts pathways, whilst behaviour is ongoing. There is thus no time for neural plasticity to kick in, no time for learning to occur or for another area to take over the role. Injecting an agonist of GABA into the substantia nigra of a trained monkey whilst it is fixating on a point, results in the monkey being unable to hold steady the eye movement. In other words the eye muscles cannot generate the saccades needed to keep the monkey's fovea focused on the point of interest. The gaze drifts away from the fixed point.

The gaze soon jumps back again to the point of interest as the effect of the agonist wears off. This is because the superior colliculus receives many other inputs including excitatory inputs from the frontal eye fields (the frontal lobes are implicated in the planning of movement). In this experiment the inputs from the frontal lobes are not affected. Also the normal balance of activity in the basal ganglia's internal circuits between the dopaminergic and GABAergic pathways is soon restored. However, it is clear that maintaining the inhibitory output from the substantia nigra has had an immediate effect on the muscles of the eye: the eye position cannot be held steady because the saccadic movements are not generated. To use the gate analogy again – the 'gate' stays shut.

Does this gating mechanism operate in other motor control systems? It seems that it does. Experiments that inject the GABAergic agonist into the globus pallidus result in the monkey being unable to hold a hand steady in a fixed position. The hand drifts away from the desired position until the monkey sees that it is in the wrong place and shifts it back.

Lesions to the basal ganglia have wide-reaching effects on movement control. As well as problems associated with initiation of movement, patients with Parkinson's disease have what is described as *bradykinesia*, which is an overall poverty of movement (too little activity). This is consistent with the findings above because individuals with Parkinson's disease have an increased GABAergic output so there is a permanent 'brake' or 'gate' operating on the pathway from the thalamus to the motor cortex. However, the symptoms of Parkinson's disease are more widespread than those obtained by manipulating GABAergic output. This is not unexpected when you remember that, for these patients, problems stem from loss of dopaminergic cells and thus lowered dopamine output, so symptoms also derive from effects on other pathways within the basal ganglia and between the basal ganglia and other structures. There are many circuits within the basal ganglia and we are a long way from understanding all of their functions. In this section we have examined the effects of altering the output from the basal ganglia, we have not investigated internal circuits and how they may operate to bring about the changes in output. Clinical observations on patients with Parkinson's disease indicate that basal ganglia do not simply select between competing motor behaviours but have a more global effect on the way that movements are controlled. The normal smooth and natural way that we move our bodies or hold them at rest is lost to the Parkinson's disease sufferer.

To return to the point made in the introduction, it is thought that the basal ganglia make a more important contribution to the control of movements that are

self-generated or internally guided as opposed to those movements that are cued by an external stimulus. The role of the basal ganglia is critical when you serve in a game of tennis, less so when you return the serve. This is one of the many topics being actively researched as we attempt to understand the roles of the basal ganglia and thereby improve the prognosis for individuals who suffer from movement disorders stemming from basal ganglia dysfunctions.

As we said at the beginning of this section, in the 17th century it was thought that the basal ganglia were the part of the brain that controlled movement directly but this changed over the next two centuries as the importance of the motor cortex was 'discovered'. In the next section we will see how this came about.

Summary of Section 3.2

Anatomical pathways link the basal ganglia and motor cortex in a loop. The normal inhibitory GABAergic output from the basal ganglia can be interrupted as a consequence of input from the motor cortex and thalamus. The removal of inhibitory signals originating from the basal ganglia allows motor activity to occur. If the inhibitory signals are artificially maintained by, for example, an injection of a GABA agonist, movement is blocked.

3.3   The cerebral cortex and voluntary movement

3.3.1   Physiological evidence for the role of the motor cortex

In the late 19th century it was discovered that electrical stimulation of certain areas of the cerebral cortex of monkeys and dogs produced movement on the opposite side of the body. In the mid 20th century, the neurosurgeon Wilder Penfield investigated these motor areas in the human cortex. This was done during operations to cure intractable epilepsy, which required the cortex to be exposed. Penfield and colleagues found that the movements produced by the electrical stimulation, which tended to be simple movements of single joints, depended on the precise site of stimulation. From repeated observations, they were able to construct a map of the human motor cortex showing which body part moved when a given part of the cortex was stimulated (Figure 3.4). One interesting aspect of this map is that the representation of the body in the motor cortex is orderly – adjacent parts on the body are represented in adjacent parts of the cortex. This ordered organization is known as **somatotopy** (see also Book 1, Section 3.4.6).

Intracellular recordings using microelectrodes (Book 3, Section 2.4.1) from a single cortical neuron from the hand region of the motor cortex can be made while a monkey performs voluntary movement. Experiments of this type have shown cortical activity to precede activity in the muscles. The cortical neuron's firing rate increases before the increase in the hand muscle's electromyography (Box 2.1 and Figure 3.5).

◈   Do the experimental data provide good evidence that the motor cortex initiates voluntary movement?

◆   No, the data do not show that the cortical activity actually causes (or even helps cause) the muscle activity, just that it precedes it. (In Section 3.2 we noted that the neurons in the superior colliculi fire prior to the initiation of a saccade but we did not suggest that the superior colliculi initiated the movement.)

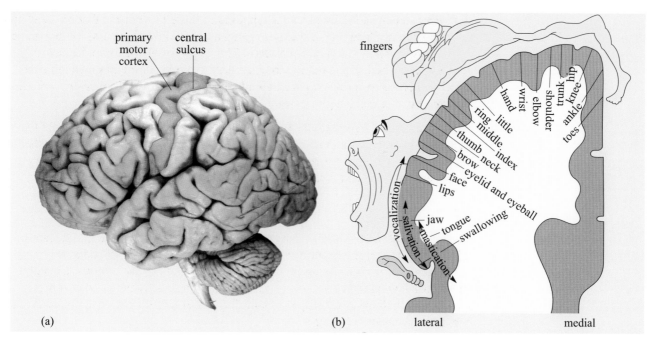

Figure 3.4 (a) The motor cortex occupies the fold, or gyrus, immediately in front of (anterior to) the central sulcus. (b) Representation of the various body parts in the motor cortex. Although the representation is somatotopic (adjacent parts of the body are represented in adjacent parts of the cortex), it is clear that it is not proportional. For example the whole of the trunk is represented in a small part of the motor cortex whereas the fingers and hand are represented in a large part. It should be noted that more recent and detailed mapping studies of the motor cortex reveal that the type of representation shown here, while broadly correct, is something of a simplification. In fact, muscle groups seem each to be represented at many different sites within the cortex. The significance of this is not yet clear.

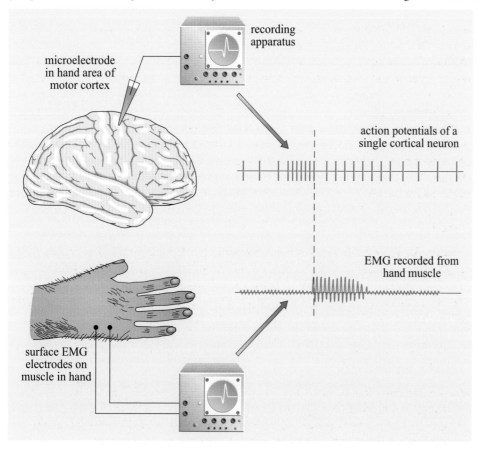

Figure 3.5 During voluntary activation of a hand muscle, a single neuron, found in the hand area of the motor cortex, always increases its firing rate before the onset of EMG activity in the muscle. Note that the recording from the cortical neuron is intracellular, a microelectrode having been manoeuvred until it pierces a single cell. Thus the trace shows the action potentials of just this one cell. In contrast, the muscle EMG is an extracellular recording of the combined effect of action potentials in many muscle fibres, as detected on the skin overlying the muscle (see Box 2.1 on electromyography).

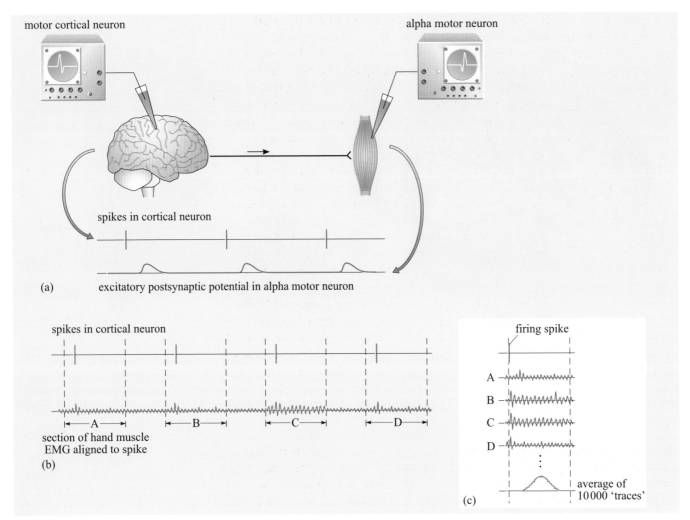

Figure 3.6   (a) If it were possible to record from a motor cortical neuron and an alpha motor neuron (in the spinal cord) with which the cortical neuron was thought to synapse, and to eradicate all other synaptic input to the motor neuron, you would expect each spike (action potential) in the cortical neuron to be followed by an EPSP (or IPSP) in the alpha motor neuron. This would be very good evidence for the existence of the putative synaptic connection. However, since this is not possible, evidence for a direct synaptic connection must be sought through less direct methods. One such method is spike-triggered averaging, as shown in (b). (b) The spikes recorded from a neuron in the hand region of the motor cortex are used to select portions of the EMG signal recorded from a hand muscle that the cortical neuron is thought to influence (i.e. it is thought to synapse with some of the muscle's alpha motor neurons). Some 10 000 or more such portions are averaged. If there were no synaptic connection between the cortical neuron and the muscle's motor neurons, the averaged trace would be expected to be flat and featureless because the criterion used to select each section would in fact have no relation to that section. Over a large number of such sections, the pseudorandom peaks and troughs of the EMG signal would average out to approximately zero. If however a synaptic connection exists, its influence will contribute to the EMG trace at the same point in each selected portion and will therefore alone 'survive' the averaging process, getting stronger as the rest of the trace tends towards zero. Thus the averaging process has the effect of bringing the signal that we are looking for out of the surrounding noise, as shown in (c).

The time-locking of this cortical activity to the muscle EMG may be because it is essential to some other aspect of the movement, for example your awareness of it. Another part of the brain altogether could be responsible for activating the muscles. This illustrates just how careful you have to be when interpreting experimental data.

In fact, by using an ingenious technique called **spike-triggered averaging**, it has been possible to demonstrate that motor cortical activity is actually instrumental in producing the muscle activation of voluntary movement. The spikes referred to are the action potentials in the cortical neuron.

You might like to reread Book 3, Section 2.4.1 where event-related potentials were discussed and the technique of averaging was described. Spike-triggered averaging works in an analogous way and as follows. If the cortical neuron (from which the recording is being made) makes an excitatory synapse onto one of the alpha motor neurons of the muscle then every time the cortical neuron fires, it will produce an excitatory postsynaptic potential (EPSP) in this motor neuron (Figure 3.6a). There will be many other neurons synapsing onto this motor neuron, some of which will have excitatory effects and some of which will have inhibitory effects. Whether or not the motor neuron fires, or how fast it fires, will depend on the sum of all of these inputs. It is important to bear in mind that the many EPSPs and inhibitory postsynaptic potentials (IPSPs) occurring in the motor neuron are uncorrelated and appear to occur randomly in time. It follows that, on average, the motor neuron will be more likely to fire during one of the EPSPs produced by the cortical neuron (or any other excitatory input) than at other times. This is a rather subtle point which is worth thinking carefully about. The spikes of the cortical neuron are used as time markers to select portions of the EMG signal to average (Figure 3.6b). When sufficient (10 000 or more) such portions are averaged, a peak is found in the EMG signal (muscle activity) *after* the timing spike (cortical neuron activity) (Figure 3.6c). The only reasonable explanation for this is that the cortical neuron has an excitatory effect on some of the alpha motor neurons of the muscle in question. In other words it contributes to or helps cause the movement.

3.3.2 Anatomical connections between the motor cortex and spinal cord

Having established a role for the motor cortex in initiating voluntary movement, we will remind ourselves of the route through the CNS that the signals take. (This was first described in Book 1, Section 3.4.6.) The output cells of the motor cortex send signals either via direct projections to other parts of the cortex or via the pyramidal tract that passes by way of the internal capsule down to the brainstem and spinal cord (Figure 3.7; see also Book 1, Figure 3.28).

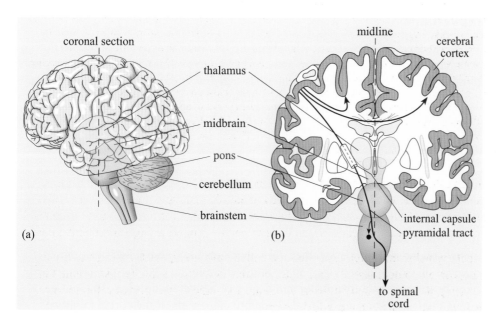

Figure 3.7 (a) Simplified diagram of the human brain viewed from the side showing the brainstem, thalamus and cerebellum. (b) Outputs from an area of cortex travel either to another part of the cortex (in the same or other hemisphere), or to the brainstem and spinal cord via the internal capsule and pyramidal tract. Those bypassing the brainstem continue along the pyramidal tract, most crossing the midline at the level of the medulla before passing into the spinal cord.

One estimate suggests that there are about 1 000 000 fibres in the human pyramidal tract (although not all of these arise from the motor cortex).

Axons travelling only as far as the brainstem synapse there with neurons in the various brainstem nuclei, many of which in turn send projections down into the spinal cord. The others bypass the brainstem completely and continue along the pyramidal tract down into the spinal cord. These are termed corticospinal fibres.

In primates, but not other mammals, some of the corticospinal fibres make direct synaptic contact with spinal alpha motor neurons that innervate the muscles of the hands. (It is these direct connections that produce the results seen in spike-triggered averaging experiments.) As these direct connections are only found in primates, we might guess that they have something to do with our highly developed ability to manipulate objects, for example tools, with our hands.

Other corticospinal fibres do not synapse directly onto motor neurons but onto a variety of interneurons. We have met one of these types of interneuron in our discussion of the spinal circuitry underlying the coordination of muscles about a single joint. We saw there how fibres descending from the brain synapse with these interneurons, modulating the activity of the spinal circuitry. Many of these descending fibres will be corticospinal fibres. Other types of interneuron that are under the direct influence of the motor cortex participate in more extensive and complicated circuitry, possibly involving simultaneous control of movement at several joints, for example the reaching movements we make with our arms.

Whether a corticospinal fibre synapses directly with alpha motor neurons or just with interneurons, it always synapses with a large number of them. Just as incoming spindle afferents branch very extensively within the spinal cord, descending corticospinal fibres do exactly the same and synapse with a large number of spinal neurons. Furthermore, anatomical techniques in which a tracer is injected into a single corticospinal fibre have shown that these fibres not only synapse with motor neurons controlling a single muscle, but also with motor neurons controlling other muscles, and sometimes with muscles in different limbs.

3.3.3 The role of the motor cortex in voluntary movement

We have seen that motor cortical neurons are involved in activating muscles during voluntary movement (courtesy of spike-triggered averaging) and that, even in the most direct connections that these neurons make with the spinal cord, they synapse with neurons controlling more than one muscle. These are a couple of useful pieces of information but they do not really tell us what the motor cortex does, i.e. what its role is in the control of voluntary movement.

Consider the problem for a moment in relation to the situation of reaching for something that you can see and must direct your movement towards rather than our previous example of waving to granny. In order to reach for a cup of tea, many muscles have to be activated in a precisely defined order and to a precisely defined degree. (You will see a little later just how complicated and critical this process is.) If you make such a reaching movement you will probably notice that your shoulder, elbow and wrist all move together. How much each of these joints must move depends on exactly where the cup is. Somewhere in the CNS the muscles needed must be selected, and their order and degree of activation decided. The motor cortex might be doing all of this, but equally other parts of the cortex might be

doing it and then simply passing on the output via the motor cortex, making it little more than a glorified relay station. Or, more likely, the job might be shared around, with the motor cortex doing just a part of the work. Any of these scenarios would be sufficient to explain the result of the spike-triggered averaging experiments described above.

We saw in our discussion of long-latency reflexes that the motor cortex appears to be involved in channelling signals from the receptors (i.e. muscle spindles) in one group of muscles into other groups of muscles, producing useful responses anywhere in the musculature at reflex latency and according to the prevailing conditions. Maybe then part of its role in voluntary movement control is some sort of analogous switching or routing function.

◆   Would the motor cortex be likely to control individual muscles?

◆   No, because each of its output cells appears to be connected to more than one muscle.

The use of spike-triggered averaging, extended to look at several muscles, has confirmed this to be the case. So the motor cortex does *not* control single muscles. We can at least be clear about that.

We noted that stimulating the motor cortex electrically produces simple movements at one joint, so maybe its role is to control some aspect of single joint movement. However, there are other regions of the cerebral cortex, known as the premotor and supplementary motor areas, where electrical stimulation also evokes movement, but the movements produced are more complex, typically involving several joints. Stimulation in these areas can evoke naturalistic reaching movements. These regions are known to send projections to the motor cortex. So perhaps they put together or plan a complex movement like reaching and then get the motor cortex to deal with the details of producing the individual joint movements required. One interesting piece of evidence that the supplementary motor area (SMA) is involved in planning movements comes from PET studies, which show that the SMA is active not only when participants make movements, but also when they just imagine making them. The motor cortex on the other hand is only active when the movement is actually executed.

A further study of interest in discriminating between the activities of these different motor areas required participants to learn and then repeat a complicated sequence of finger movements. Once they were engaged in this task, transcranial magnetic stimulation (TMS; see Book 3, Section 2.4.1) was applied above the hand region on the primary motor cortex. Immediately the fingers 'misbehaved' – either the 'wrong' one moved or nothing happened. The participants reported a loss of control over the movements of their fingers. By contrast, when the TMS was moved to above the SMA there was a slight delay before any effect was noticed, then the sequence was disrupted and again the 'wrong' fingers moved. This time the participant's *perception* of what had happened was different. They felt that they had 'lost the plot', i.e. they had suddenly forgotten the sequence, rather than that they knew what they wanted to do but had lost control.

The SMA has extensive connections with the prefrontal cortex as well as with the primary motor cortex and the basal ganglia. Thus the plans created in the SMA can be influenced by emotions and memories and accessed by the basal ganglia. These pathways, known as the ventromedial motor pathway (because of their location),

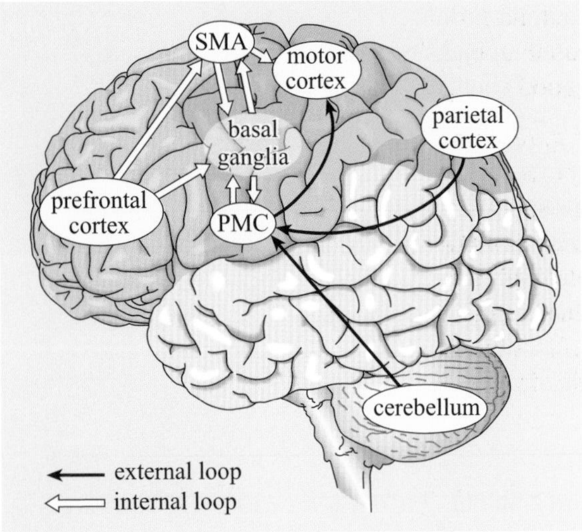

Figure 3.8   The ventromedial motor pathway, indicated by white arrows, is active when movements are internally guided. Note: PMC is the premotor cortex; SMA is the supplementary motor area.

shown schematically in Figure 3.8, form an *internal loop* that Goldberg (1985) suggests is of major importance when an action is internally guided. (You may remember in Section 3.2 that we said the basal ganglia were thought to be more important when movements are self-generated.)

The black arrows on Figure 3.8 show another set of pathways termed the *external loop*. In this case the motor cortex receives input from the premotor cortex (PMC) where information from the parietal cortex and cerebellum is integrated. We will be finding out more about the cerebellum in Section 3.4, but you already know from your study of Book 1 that these pathways will be bringing a rich sensory input to inform the planning of motor activity (hence the designation 'external' loop).

We now have a model for the control of our pianist's fingers and can imagine the integration of emotion with carefully learned finger movements, generating a plan in the SMA that is passed to motor cortex. Commands are transmitted down the corticospinal pathway. The alpha motor neurons cause the muscles to contract and the surfaces of the fingers to strike the keys with just the right force to create the sounds that the pianist imagined as the plan unfolded in the SMA. This hierarchical model, which was also proposed in Book 1, Section 3.4.6 is a nice idea (and it looks like there is some truth in it), but can we use it to explain all movements?

If we return for a moment to the task we considered at the beginning of this section, the reaching movement, we immediately hit a snag with our model. Monkeys lacking a motor cortex can still make reaching movements. In fact they can still do almost everything. Humans with stroke damage to the motor cortex are also still able to move. This alerts us to a new subtlety. Very often, when some part of the motor system is destroyed no obvious deficits are produced. Usually, the reason for this is that a number of parts of the system can all do a given job. The system is said to exhibit *redundancy*. Normally, these various parts will contribute to the overall output in different ways, according to the task and the circumstances. But when one of these parts ceases to function, the others can more or less take over. Sometimes they might need a week or two to get the hang of it, but after that few obvious deficits are to be seen. In this case it turns out that premotor and supplementary motor areas, as well as projecting to the motor cortex, also project to the spinal cord and the brainstem nuclei (just as the motor cortex does). When the motor cortex is not present, these other motor areas can just about handle most things.

It is possible to imagine how this sort of 'belt and braces' arrangement could help an injured animal to survive, and we might assume that this is why the motor systems have come to exhibit so much redundancy. The reality, however, may be a little less straightforward. It seems that, through the course of evolution, increasingly sophisticated motor control systems, rather than replacing, have been added to what was already there. By the time you get to a human being you have a baffling array of systems, partly working in parallel, partly working in some sort of hierarchy, and together often exhibiting a high degree of redundancy. Rather than seeing this as some wonderfully elusive, finely tuned product of natural selection, it

is tempting to see it all as a bit of a mess. As Darwin himself pointed out, natural selection does not produce perfect organisms, just ones that are 'good enough'. We may be a bit of a mess, but, since we are still here, we are obviously good enough.

We have already said that humans with damage to the motor cortex, e.g. resulting from a stroke, can still move. Some movement control is, however, permanently lost. Typically, fine control of the fingers is impossible. Rather than moving individually, the fingers all move together rendering the individual clumsy at tasks requiring fine control of the hand, such as doing up buttons. Fine control of facial muscles and of speech may also be lost. In addition there may be a general deficit in the speed of voluntary movement. The appearance of these various deficits is variable because the extent of the damage resulting from a stroke varies from case to case.

3.3.4   Controlling multijoint movement: reaction forces in reaching

We have already said that when you reach for a cup of tea, your shoulder, elbow and wrist all move together. How much each of these joints must move depends on exactly where the cup is. So we might imagine that the brain's task is to work out how much each joint needs to move and then to get the movements to happen. This is very much more involved than you might at first think.

One problem is that movement at one joint will, in general, cause movement at other joints.

You can readily demonstrate this to yourself by carrying out Activity 3.1.

Activity 3.1

Hold out your arm in front of you with your palm facing upwards and the elbow almost fully extended (almost straight). If you now flex (bend) the elbow *quickly* you will note that the shoulder joint also moves, briefly taking the upper arm downwards (Figure 3.9).

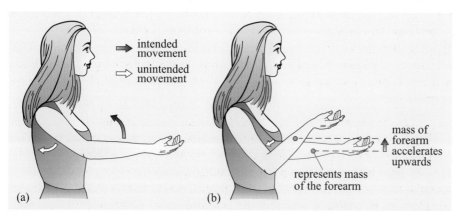

Figure 3.9   (a) Rapid flexion of the elbow leads to involuntary movement at the shoulder. (b) When the elbow is flexed, the upper arm exerts an upward force on the forearm resulting in the forearm's mass being accelerated upwards. This gives rise to a downwards reaction force on the upper arm, resulting in movement of the shoulder.

When you carried out Activity 3.1 there was movement at the shoulder that you did not intend to make. This movement arises from a property of all physical systems – whenever you exert a force on something, it exerts a force back on you. This **reaction force** is equal in magnitude to the force you exert, but opposite in direction. This principle is enshrined in Newton's third law of motion, 'To every action there is an equal and opposite reaction.' In the case of the elbow flexion movement we are considering, the biceps contraction produces a force which accelerates the forearm upwards. The forearm thus produces a reaction force downwards, which acts on the upper arm, because this is what is pushing the forearm upwards. It is this reaction force that produces the downward motion at the shoulder that you observe (Figure 3.9b).

The shoulder movement that you see occurs despite the fact that, when you flex your elbow in this way, your shoulder muscles are automatically being brought into action to stabilize the shoulder and stop it moving. In other words your CNS 'knows' about the problem and takes what steps it can to minimize the unwanted movement. But it cannot completely eradicate it because the reaction force produced by a quick movement, although brief, is very large and muscles cannot be made sufficiently stiff to resist such large forces. If the shoulder was not stabilized in this way, rapid flexion of the elbow would lead equally to rapid flexion of the shoulder and you would end up almost elbowing yourself in the ribs.

Many neuroscientists now think that the presence of reaction phenomena constitutes the greatest challenge to the CNS in controlling our everyday movement. It is the reaction forces that make the job really difficult. Thus the problem of controlling many joints is not simply that of controlling a single joint, multiplied by the number of joints involved. Since virtually all of the movements we make in everyday life involve the simultaneous control of multiple joints, our CNS has constantly to take reaction forces into account. We will now consider the implications of this in the act of reaching.

When you make a reaching movement, your hand appears to move in approximately a straight line – try it! We don't usually move our hands in a perfectly straight line, but we do get very close. Consider the problem with the help of Figure 3.10. If you want to take the finger tips from A to B along a straight-line path you have to move the three joints involved (shoulder, elbow and wrist) together. For example it would be no good just opening up the elbow joint first because this would take the fingertips way off course, as shown in Figure 3.10. The movements of joints need to be coordinated.

With the help of a little geometry and head-scratching we may be able to work out how the three joints might move together in order to produce the straight-line path for the fingertips. You may have noticed that there is no unique solution to this problem. In fact there is an infinite number of solutions. We will just gloss over this point here, but it is a real problem. How does the CNS choose which solution to use? Let's say that the CNS 'knows its geometry' too, so it can also work this out. So far so good. But now it has to work out how to produce these movements with the muscles, and this is where the problems really begin. One of these problems (and it is only one of them) is the presence of reaction forces. As the CNS opens out (extends) the elbow joint, the movement of the forearm will cause the shoulder and wrist joints to move.

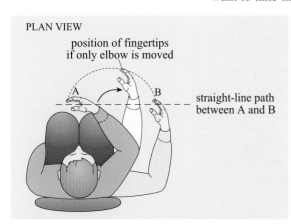

PLAN VIEW

position of fingertips if only elbow is moved

A   B

straight-line path between A and B

Figure 3.10   To take the fingertips from A to B in a straight-line path requires the simultaneous movement of all three joints (shoulder, elbow and wrist). Movement of the elbow alone to its position where the fingertips are at B results in a large deviation from the straight-line path.

So the CNS has to add compensation for these effects into the commands that it already needs to send to the shoulder and wrist muscles in order to get them to move at the right time and by the right amount.

It is already starting to seem complicated, but it just gets worse and worse. Movement at the shoulder will cause movement of the elbow and wrist. This too must be compensated for. In general, movement anywhere causes movement everywhere else, and everything has to be compensated for if an even vaguely straight-line path is to result. Not only that, but everything is crucially dependent on the overall speed of the movement. Reaction forces increase in size with increase in the speed at which the joints are moving. So all of the compensations will be different for even a slightly different movement speed. In fact, the calculations are so horrendously difficult that very few people believe that the CNS can possibly do them. It doesn't even have very long to do them. When you fancy another sip of tea, you cannot wait around for an hour or so while your brain 'crunches numbers'. But the fact remains that we can and do move our hands in approximately straight-line paths. So how on earth do we do it?

Recent research suggests that it is all a bit of a 'bodge' job. Basically, what seems to happen is that the CNS launches the movement with a set of commands to the muscles that are only approximately correct. They are a 'best guess' at what is required. The CNS then immediately starts to monitor the movement as it evolves and makes corrections to it 'on the fly'. In this way it produces a reasonable approximation of a straight-line path. As Darwin said, 'not perfect, but good enough.'

The evidence for this comes from studies in which participants were asked to make reaching movements similar to the one depicted in Figure 3.10. A range of different target positions were used. In some studies, the muscle activations required to start the movement in the correct direction for each target position were worked out using a computer. The muscle activations actually used by the participants when reaching to each of these target positions were then recorded using surface EMG. Comparison with the computed predictions showed that participants frequently did not start the movements with the 'correct' muscle activations. For certain target locations they did not even start with the 'correct' set of muscles.

In other studies, normal individuals were compared with individuals who had no functional sensory afferent fibres. (This latter state is known as deafferentation.) The reaching movements of both groups started by deviating from a straight-line path, but whereas the normal participants quickly corrected for the deviation, the deafferented participants did not. This suggests that proprioception is used in making ongoing corrections to the movement once it has begun.

Another research technique involved adding weights to one of the arm segments. This changes the reaction forces produced when that segment is moved and so should change the muscle activations used to initiate a reaching movement. However, participants did not make appropriate changes to the initial muscle activations, relying instead on correcting the movement once it had begun. This behaviour, which persisted despite practice with the weighted arm, resulted in greater deviations from the straight-line path.

Taken together, these results suggest that the problem of working out in advance the muscle activations required to produce a straight-line arm movement is in fact too difficult. What the CNS is doing instead is using a mixture of feedforward and

feedback control. The arm movement is monitored as it occurs using proprioceptors, and deviations from the intended trajectory are corrected (feedback). But until the arm movement is underway there is nothing to monitor and correct, so the whole thing has to be initiated with a set of muscle commands that are worked out in advance (feedforward). Of course, the closer these are to what is actually required, the better, because this will necessitate less correction. But the presence of a correcting mechanism will allow significant errors in this initial estimate.

Having read about all of this complexity, try making another straight-line reaching movement. It seems impossible to believe that it could be as difficult as we have been making out. It just seems so easy to do. However, confirmation that it really is anything but easy comes from studies on people who, through disease, have lost the ability to move their arms in this controlled fashion. Early in the next section we look at some of these data.

Summary of Section 3.3

The artificial stimulation of specific areas of the motor cortex results in predictable movements being generated. Spike-triggered averaging confirms that motor cortical activity produces these movements. Motor cortical neurons do not synapse directly with alpha motor neurons except in the primate hand, nor do they control individual muscles. They may, however, control some aspects of single joint movement on the instructions from premotor and supplementary motor areas that plan the overall ongoing body movements. By looking into whole body movements we become aware of the issue of reaction forces. Taking account of these forces to plan the sequencing and coordination of muscle activity requires such complex computation that it is doubtful whether the detail could be planned in advance. It seems more likely that the initial motor commands are a feedforward package that can be refined by muscle adjustments that are made from moment to moment based on proprioceptive feedback.

3.4   The cerebellum

3.4.1   The cerebellum: controlling and learning sequences of movements

The cerebellum, although constituting only about 10% of total brain volume, contains more neurons than the whole of the rest of the brain put together. There are a number of distinct parts to the cerebellum, each having different connections to the rest of the brain. Look again at Figure 3.8 and you will see how the cerebellum is connected to the motor cortex through the premotor cortex (PMC). The particular cerebellar area that does this is called the *neocerebellum*. All its output is sent via the thalamus (not shown on Figure 3.8). Projections are made to prefrontal cortex and primary motor cortex as well as to PMC. The major input to the neocerebellum is from the cerebral cortex, especially the parietal and frontal lobes. Another area of the cerebellum (*spinocerebellum*) mainly sends output to the spinal cord and nuclei of the extrapyramidal system, i.e. all descending motor pathways except the corticospinal (or pyramidal) tract. It receives sensory input from the spinal cord in addition to visual and auditory sources. The *vestibulocerebellum* receives information from, and projects to, the vestibular system (Figure 3.11). We will examine the functioning of this system in the next section.

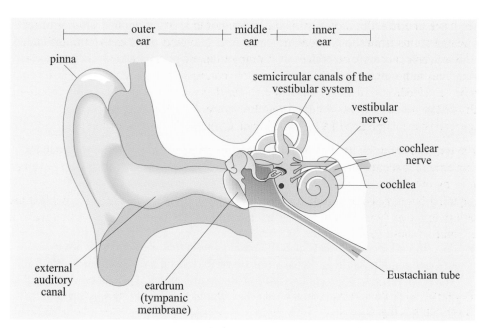

Throughout the whole of the cerebellum, neurons are connected together in a very similar and relatively simple repeating pattern as shown in Figure 1.26b. This suggests that each part of the cerebellum might carry out the same basic function, but applied to different brain systems because of the different connections. The highly regular and repetitive neuronal structure appears to be suited to the generation or representation of temporal patterns of neuronal activity and, by implication, to the sequencing of muscular contractions. We know that the cerebellum is involved in the control of movement and balance because when it is damaged, through disease or trauma, deficits appear in movement and/or balance control.

For example, as we have been discussing, when a healthy individual makes a reaching movement, their hand moves reasonably directly to its target. When, however, someone with cerebellar dysfunction (for example Friedereich's ataxia, a degenerative condition in which input to the cerebellum is disrupted) attempts the same thing, the hand typically moves erratically and indirectly. The control system is still working to some extent (the hand ends up at least close to the target), but it is very far from working properly. The arm veers and swerves seemingly out of control. In many cases the hand starts to oscillate violently as the target is approached. This *intention tremor* is often contrasted with a *rest tremor* found in Parkinson's disease (see Section 1.6.4).

So damage to the cerebellum results in poor coordination and a lack of precision in movement. A patient with damage to the right lobe of the cerebellum reported, 'The movements of my left arm are done subconsciously, but I have to think out each movement of the right arm.' The cerebellum, unlike the motor cortex, influences the muscles on the ipsilateral (same) side of the body.

Sir John Eccles (one of Sherrington's pupils), who spent much of his research career studying the cerebellum, suggested that cortical centres give general commands to carry out movement, leaving the computation and execution to subcortical, notably cerebellar, mechanisms. One aspect of behaviour to which the cerebellum has long been known to make a contribution is in the production of *ballistic* responses. Ballistic responses are learned sequences of behaviour that are carried out too fast for the brain to use any sensory feedback from the muscles to

sequence and structure. That is, a ballistic response is 'programmed' as a temporal sequence of muscular movements. Examples of ballistic sequences are the so-called 'instinctively' accurate responses of champion tennis players and cricketers that are acquired with much practice.

◆ Do you think pianists use ballistic movements?

◆ Obviously not whilst learning! But as soon as they are able to perform those spectacular high-speed passages beloved by concert pianists they will be using ballistic movements.

◆ Do you think that someone with Parkinson's disease will be able to use ballistic movement?

◆ Yes. In Parkinson's disease it is the basal ganglia that are damaged, not the cerebellum. (In fact it is a characteristic of Parkinson's disease that the sufferer can often respond appropriately with ballistic movement. For example, if a ball is hurled at them they can catch it, but they would find it exceedingly difficult to throw the ball back.)

The ability to produce ballistic sequences of muscle control is important in sustaining movement without involving the CNS in excessive levels of computation, which would be necessary if the sensory consequences of every muscle movement had to be processed before the next was initiated. In this context, the cerebellum has been implicated in motor learning, i.e. in learning sequences of muscle movement so that the activity becomes 'automatic'.

The cerebellum is clearly involved in the control of movement and in learning sequences of movements. In turn, this depends on being able to compute and control the timing of each movement. But how does the cerebellum do this? We do not exactly know. However, as with the motor cortex, there are a number of findings which offer tantalizing glimpses. We will have a look here at just one of these, the cerebellum's involvement in the **vestibular ocular reflex (VOR)**, which is an important aspect of eye movement control. We will then discuss to what extent this might give us clues as to the cerebellum's general role in movement control.

3.4.2 The vestibular ocular reflex

Activity 3.2

Hold up an index finger about 30 cm in front of your face and begin to move it slowly from side to side through about 30 cm, keeping your gaze on it so that it remains in focus (move just your eyes, not your head). Now gradually speed up the side-to-side movement. You will get to a point where you can no longer keep the finger in focus. Note the approximate speed of movement at which this happens. Now hold up the finger again and this time, keeping the finger still, move your head from side to side while looking at the finger. Increase the speed of movement until you can no longer keep the finger in focus.

You should find that you can keep the finger focused at much faster movement speeds when moving your head rather than your finger.

In Activity 3.2, you were keeping your eyes on your finger whilst either the finger or the head was in motion. The movement of the eyes in the orbits is similar in both conditions. In other words the same muscles, the extra-ocular muscles, are being activated in broadly the same way. The reason for the discrepancy in the results you observed when carrying out Activity 3.2 is that different *control* mechanisms are being used in the two conditions. They may both activate the same muscles in a similar way, but that is where the similarity ends. Both mechanisms exist just in order to control eye movements.

Head motion (angular acceleration) is picked up by the semicircular canals of the vestibular system of the inner ear (see Figure 3.11) and, via a simple and (therefore) fast neural circuit, is used to activate the extra-ocular muscles and drive the eyes in the opposite direction to the head motion (Figure 3.12). This mechanism is the vestibular ocular reflex. The *gain* of this pathway (i.e. how much eye movement is produced for a given head movement) is exactly set such that the images on the retinas remain stable. In other words, the movement of the eyes is just enough to compensate for the movement of the head. This is why the world does not appear to move whenever you move your head. Disease of the vestibular system can lead to abnormal function of this reflex with sufferers experiencing the world 'swimming around' whenever they move their heads. It goes without saying that this is extremely debilitating.

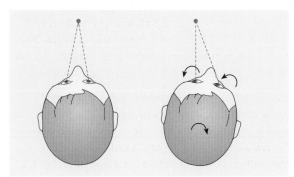

Figure 3.12   Rotation of the head stimulates the semicircular canals of the vestibular apparatus and, via the pathway of the vestibular ocular reflex, leads to counter-rotation of the eyes such that the image on the retinas is held stable. Arrows indicate direction of movement.

The VOR is of course not available in Activity 3.2 when the head is held still and the finger is moved. Here we rely on a different control system in different parts of the brain. When the eyes need to follow a moving object they are said to track or pursue the object; the eye movements produced are described as **smooth pursuit**. If the eyes are following an object which suddenly and unpredictably changes direction, there is a delay between the change in the object's and the eyes' direction of movement.

When you watch a moving object, your eyes follow or pursue it in an attempt to keep its image on the fovea. If the object moves predictably, for example with constant velocity, the smooth pursuit mechanism can achieve this. If, however, the object suddenly changes direction, there is a delay before the eyes catch up with, and once again track, its movement. The presence of the delay reveals that smooth pursuit is in part a feedback mechanism. However, the absence of any delay when tracking an object moving at constant velocity reveals that it also works predictively. The speed and direction of the object is immediately noted and the CNS begins to move the eyes at this speed and direction, effectively assuming that the object will continue to move in this way. (If such a predictive mode of control were not used, the movement of the eyes would lag behind that of the object by a constant amount.)

This is another example of the inevitable delay associated with a feedback control system, which is partly what the smooth pursuit system is. Only partly though. Like the systems controlling reaching movements (Section 3.3.4) and stretch responses in muscles (Section 2.10.1), the smooth pursuit mechanism uses prediction to help get around feedback delays. When faced with an object that the CNS 'realizes' is moving in a predictable path (for example constant speed and direction), it begins to move the eyes through this predictable path, anticipating rather than following the object's motion. This can reduce the lag between object and eye movement approximately to zero. However, despite this advanced predictive ability, the smooth pursuit system still cannot function at the speed of the VOR.

The VOR is fast because there are very few synapses between sense organ and effector (see below). But the reason that it can be this simple is that it is effectively a feedforward system. When it receives an input it immediately produces an output, which it in effect 'assumes' to be correct. It 'throws' a package of commands at the extra-ocular muscles with complete confidence that they will produce the required eye movement.

◆ What are the problems for this feedforward system if, for example, you are growing?

◆ As you grow, your head and your eyes change shape and get bigger, as do your muscles, including the extra-ocular muscles.

◆ How can the gain of the VOR continue to be appropriate in the face of all of these changes?

◆ The answer is that it cannot. The gain of the VOR has to adjust, and this is where the cerebellum comes in.

Without the VOR, the images on your retina would move by a certain fixed amount for a given head movement. It is this relationship to which your VOR is 'calibrated'. It is possible, using prisms, to make spectacles that change this relationship, for example they might increase the movement of the image on the retina for a given head movement. Wearing such spectacles is an extremely strange and unpleasant experience. Every time you move your head the world moves. In fact, if you wear glasses, you might have had similar albeit less dramatic experiences. Changing your glasses prescription, walking around without your glasses on, or changing from contact lenses to spectacles at the end of the day can all produce a strange 'swishing about' of the world as you move. This is because any lens will change slightly the relationship between head motion and retinal image motion.

Thankfully for those of us who are visually challenged, this effect is short-lived. It typically goes away in minutes. This is also the case with the prism spectacles, although the adaptation can take much longer because the change they produce can be much greater. But if you wear them for long enough, everything seems to get back to more or less normal. It must be the case then that the VOR is now working at a different gain, i.e. producing a larger or smaller movement of the eyes in response to a given movement of the head. It has adapted. The crucial observation for us here is that an intact cerebellum is essential to this ability to adapt. Cerebellar dysfunction can leave a person unable to adapt. Thus the cerebellum is involved

here in recalibrating a feedforward control system. In a moment we will speculate as to whether this gives us a clue about the cerebellum's overall contribution to movement control. But first we will have a look at the neural circuit behind the adaptation of the VOR.

In the most direct pathway, a vestibular afferent arising in one of the semicircular canals synapses with an interneuron, which in turn synapses with a motor neuron of one of the extra-ocular muscles (Figure 3.13). In this figure we have shown only one of each type of neuron (just as we did when we considered neural circuitry in the spinal cord), but bear in mind that in reality there are hundreds of neurons. The gain of the pathway (how much eye movement is produced for a given head movement) depends on:

•   the way in which all of these neurons are connected. For example, if the vestibular afferents branch extensively, each influencing many motor neurons, a small input could produce a large output (this is an example of divergence – see Section 1.6.2);

•   the strength, or efficacy, of the synaptic connections between the neurons.

The cerebellum is connected in parallel with this pathway as shown in Figure 3.13. It is in a position to reduce the overall gain via inhibitory influences on the motor neurons, and to increase it via excitatory influences. Any changes occur as a result of an error signal arising in the retinas. If during a head movement the image on the retinas moves, or *slips*, an error signal is generated that the cerebellum uses to adjust the gain of the VOR pathway.

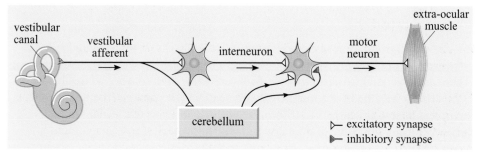

Figure 3.13   The most direct neural pathway of the vestibular ocular reflex. A vestibular afferent synapses with an interneuron, which in turn synapses with a motor neuron of an extra-ocular muscle. The cerebellum forms a side loop that can alter the gain of this reflex pathway.

This then is what happens when you put prism spectacles on. But in reality it is happening all the time. Feedforward mechanisms like the VOR are subject to constant fine-tuning. This is essential because biological systems change according to their recent history. If you go to the gym a lot you may lose weight and build muscles. A feedforward system that moved you around before you joined the gym would not work properly afterwards. Feedforward systems like the VOR seem to get the best of both worlds: the speed of a feedforward system and the self-calibrating benefits of feedback.

We noted at the beginning of this section that although the cerebellum has a number of distinct parts, each with their own inputs and outputs from and to other areas of the CNS, its neural circuitry is strikingly similar throughout. We looked at the VOR because we thought that if we knew what one part of the cerebellum did, we might know what all of it does.

In the case of the VOR the cerebellum appears to function as a tuning or calibrating system, in this case adjusting the gain of a feedforward pathway. Does this extrapolate to reaching? You will recall from our discussion of the control of reaching movements that both feedforward and feedback mechanisms are used. The feedforward component is necessary to launch the movement. However, individuals with Friedereich's ataxia make reaching movements that are apparently out of control. Although this could be due to a wildly inaccurate initiation of the movement, it seems more likely that it is also due to poor regulation of the movement once it is underway. As you move your hand in a straight line to reach a target position (as shown in Figure 3.10) the movement must be terminated *before* you are aware that you have reached the target. One way that this could be done is by timing. One hypothesis is that the cerebellum computes the amount of time that individual muscles must each work. If you have ever thrown a ball overarm you may be aware how horribly inaccurate you can be! As you swing your arm above your shoulder and then downwards it is essential to release your grip on the ball at the right moment: too soon and it sails up into the air; too late and it plummets to the ground. Research has shown that most of us get the moment of release correct 95% of the time but patients with cerebellar lesions do far worse than that. This is further evidence that the timing of movement may be a function of the cerebellum.

In general, cerebellar dysfunction appears to interfere with the timing and sequencing of movement, without regard for the particular mechanism (feedforward or feedback) being used. To this extent, its role in regulating the gain of the VOR appears to generalize to its role in movement control.

The ability to monitor ongoing motor activity and provide feedback to adjust the movement so that it matches the desired outcome as planned by the prefrontal and supplementary motor cortex means that the cerebellum also has an important role to play in the learning of new motor patterns (skills). This role too is hinted at by its involvement in changing VOR gain when circumstances change (prism spectacles). There are anecdotal stories of people with cerebellar disease who, while able to drive the car they had for a number of years before the disease, are quite unable to drive an unfamiliar car. It is as if they are not able to 'change the gain' in the pathways that control the accelerator and steering wheel.

Learning new motor skills and refining those already learned continues throughout our lives and is just one of the kinds of learning in which we indulge. Book 5 will look at learning in much more detail.

Summary of Section 3.4

The vestibular ocular reflex (VOR) enables us to hold a visual image steady whilst moving our head. It is a feedforward system that depends on there being a precisely calibrated relationship between the amount of eye movement that is needed for a given head movement. This relationship (or gain) sometimes has to be recalibrated, for example as you grow the relationship changes. Recalibration requires a feedback system. The gain on the VOR can be recalibrated, but the recalibration is not instantaneous and it can only be achieved if the cerebellum is intact. The cerebellum must therefore be the site of the feedback system. In general, damage to the cerebellum results in an inability to operate a successful feedback system for any motor activity.

Learning outcomes for Chapter 3

After studying this chapter, you should be able to:

3.1 Recognize definitions and applications of each of the terms printed in **bold** in the text.

3.2 Explain the roles of the basal ganglia and the cerebellum in movement control.

3.3 Describe the neurophysiological relationships between the motor cortex and the alpha motor neurons.

3.4 Explain why reaction forces pose a problem for the control of movement.

3.5 Relate the concepts of feedforward and feedback to motor control.

Questions for Chapter 3

Question 3.1   (Learning outcome 3.2)

In Huntington's disease the GABAergic output from the basal ganglia is reduced and the sufferer exhibits erratic and unpredictable movements. What role do you think the basal ganglia play in the selection of these movements?

Question 3.2   (Learning outcome 3.3)

Which of the following statement(s) are true and which are false?

A   Cell bodies of alpha motor neurons are located in the ventral horns of the spinal cord grey matter.

B   Voluntary (willed) movement results from interplay between descending influences from the brain and the organization of reflexes in the spinal cord.

C   The pyramidal tract is the descending pathway from the motor cortex to the brainstem motor neurons.

D   The cerebellum does not have direct connections with the motor system structures of the brain.

E   The descending pathways from the motor cortex cross over the midline at the level of the spinal cord to control the contralateral muscles.

Question 3.3   (Learning outcome 3.4)

Explain, in relation to reaction forces, why you would not expect to find a simple relationship between the number of action potentials recorded at a motor endplate and the amount of movement of a limb.

Question 3.4   (Learning outcome 3.5)

Explain the concepts of feedforward control and feedback control in relation to the movement of a limb.

Question 1.1

Description C is correct.

Question 1.2

All four statements are true.

Question 1.3

Statements A, C and E are true.

Question 1.4

Statements A, B, C, D and F are true.

Question 1.5

The statement is generally correct in that once a neuron is brought to its firing threshold it will fire an action potential. The happens because the sodium channels that mediate the action potential suddenly open, allowing sodium ions to enter the cell (flowing down their concentration and electrical gradients) which rapidly depolarize the membrane. At a membrane potential of about +20 mV the sodium channels then close, preventing further depolarization. The delayed-potassium channels now open, potassium ions leave the cell (flowing down their concentration gradient), a process which rapidly repolarizes the cell. The statement is incorrect in that it suggests that repolarization of the membrane potential is due to the sodium–potassium pump; the sodium–potassium pump 'ticks-over' at a fairly steady rate and does not fluctuate during the action potential.

Question 1.6

Statements B and C are correct.

Question 1.7

If an action potential has travelled along a portion of axon, the voltage-gated channels in the membrane of that portion need to reassume a form that allows them to open again. In other words, a refractory period must elapse. If the action potential is initiated by artificial stimulation midway along the axon, the region to either side has not been stimulated and so an action potential can spread out to either side. In a nerve cell, the generation of an action potential at one end of the axon, at the axon hillock, means that the action potential will travel in one direction only.

Question 1.8

The correct explanation is D.

Question 1.9

1 Axon (or more specifically axon terminal)
2 Synaptic vesicle
3 Presynaptic membrane
4 Synaptic cleft
5 Transmitter molecule
6 Postsynaptic membrane

Question 1.10

Action potentials arriving at the presynaptic terminal increase the permeability of the membrane to calcium ions. The resulting increased intracellular calcium ion concentration causes the neurotransmitter-filled synaptic vesicles to fuse with the presynaptic membrane and, by the process of exocytosis, to release their contents into the synaptic cleft. The neurotransmitter molecules then diffuse across the cleft and bind to receptors located on the postsynaptic membrane. The binding of neurotransmitter to the receptors alters the permeability of the postsynaptic membrane which, in turn, changes the membrane potential. Depending on the type of neurotransmitter–receptor interaction, these changes can produce EPSPs or IPSPs.

Question 1.11

A synaptic potential is a graded potential – its size is directly related to the degree of stimulation or activation. The action potential on the other hand is an all-or-nothing event.

Question 1.12

The effects would cancel out, leaving little or no change in membrane potential. The tendency of neuron 1 to depolarize is cancelled by the tendency of neuron 3 to hyperpolarize.

Question 1.13

(a) Nicotine is an agonist at nicotinic acetylcholine receptors – the receptors found at the end plate on skeletal muscle.

(b) THC is the active ingredient found in cannabis – it is an agonist at cannabinoid receptors.

(c) Haloperidol is an antagonist at dopamine receptors and has been used to alleviate the hyperkinesia associated with Huntington's disease.

Question 1.14

Stimulation of the afferent neuron in Figure 1.24 would activate two types of cell – the extensor motor neuron and an inhibitory interneuron. Activation of the extensor motor neuron causes the extensor muscles to contract. Activation of the inhibitory interneuron prevents activation of the flexor muscle by feedforward inhibition of the flexor motor neuron.

Question 2.1

Light is a physical stimulus that is transduced by photoreceptors (rods and cones of the retina). Absorption of light causes a change in the membrane potential of the photoreceptors – they hyperpolarize. The retina is responsible for the initial processing of the visual signals and the output from the retina is conveyed by the optic nerve to the brain. The optic nerve is the collection of axons of the retinal ganglion cells. Information about the visual scene is coded in the patterns of action potential firing of the retinal ganglion cells. Different cells carry information about different aspects of the visual stimulus (e.g. the face – in the lecture on face recognition referred to in the question) and these different pathways terminate in different regions of the brain.

Question 2.2

Evidence pertaining to the role of the FFA has been obtained using a variety of different techniques, experimental studies and the interpretation of the behaviour of brain-damaged individuals. This might account for some of the contradictory findings.

Question 2.3

The wing muscles of migratory birds would contain predominately fatigue-resistant units. Maximum output can be achieved by recruiting more motor units and by increasing the firing frequency of these units.

Question 2.4

A, C and D are appropriate descriptions of the muscle spindle. The structure of the muscle spindle and its relationship with the working muscle is shown in Figure 2.17. Although the muscle spindle can contract, it does not generate any significant force and does not contribute to movement of joints, therefore B is an incorrect statement.

Question 2.5

The trans-cortical hypothesis suggests that M2 reflex responses are routed from the originating muscle via the motor cortex to another muscle. In Klipper–Feil syndrome, cortical axons are thought to branch in the cervical cord, synapsing with motor neurons innervating homologous muscles in the two hands. When a Klipper–Feil individual stretches a muscle in one hand, a long-latency stretch response is recorded in both the originating muscle and in the homologous muscle in the other hand.

Question 3.1

The normal output from the basal ganglia is to the thalamus and this is at one remove from the motor cortex. The removal of the normal inhibitory output appears to 'open a gate' allowing information to flow from the thalamus to the motor cortex and making movement more likely to occur. The random nature of movements in Huntington's disease suggests that when the basal ganglia's inhibition is removed in the absence of the normal associated activity from other brain areas, the contribution of the basal ganglia is simply to make movement more likely not to select which movement should occur.

Question 3.2

A, B and D are true. C and E are false for the reasons given below:

C The pyramidal tract descends to the spinal cord motor neurons – there are no motor neurons in the brainstem.

E The pathways cross at the level of the brainstem in the structure called the pyramidal tract.

Question 3.3

Although there will be a simple relationship between the number of action potentials that arrive at the motor endplate and the number of action potentials seen in the

muscle fibre, this does not translate into a predictable amount of movement. The reason for this is that as the muscle starts to shorten and move the limb, reaction forces will oppose the movement. The extent to which they oppose the movement will depend on where the limb is when it starts to move as well as how fast it moves.

Question 3.4

In feedforward control the current sensory information, together with that recalled from memory is used to anticipate disturbances to limb dynamics and to plan appropriate muscle activation based on experience. It requires the ability to predict the consequences of different muscle activation patterns. In feedback control there is monitoring of sensory signals (generally proprioceptive and visual) which is used to provide information about limb dynamics and change muscle activation.

Chapter 1

Further reading

Kandel, E. R., Schwartz, J. H. and Jessell, T. M. (2000) *Principles of Neural Science*, 4th edn, McGraw-Hill, New York.

Carpenter, R. H. S. (2002) *Neurophysiology*, 4th edn, Arnold, London.

Bear, M. (2000) *Neuroscience: Exploring the Brain*, 1st edn, Lippincott Williams & Wilkins, New York.

Chapter 2

References

Baylis, G. C., Rolls, E. T. and Leonard, C. M. (1985) Selectivity between faces in the responses of a population of neurons in the cortex in the superior temporal sulcus of the monkey, *Brain Research*, **342**, pp. 91–102.

Gauthier, I., Skudlarski, P., Gore, J. C. and Anderson, A. W. (2000) Expertise for cars and birds recruits brain areas involved in face recognition, *Nature Neuroscience*, **3**, pp. 191–7.

Moscovitch, M., Winocur, G. and Behrmann, M. (1997) What is special about face recognition? Nineteen experiments on a person with visual object agnosia and dyslexia but normal face recognition, *Journal of Cognitive Neuroscience*, **9**, pp. 555–604.

Riddoch, M. J. and Humphreys, G. W. (1987) A case of integrative visual agnosia, *Brain*, **110**, pp. 1431–62.

Sherrington, C. S. (1933) *The Brain and its Mechanism*, Cambridge University Press, Cambridge.

Zeki, S., Watson, J. D., Lueck, C. J., Friston, K. J., Kennard, C. and Frackowiak, R. S. (1991) A direct demonstration of functional specialization in human visual cortex, *Journal of Neuroscience*, **11**, pp. 641–9.

Chapter 3

References

Goldberg, G. (1985) Supplementary motor area structure and function: review and hypothesis, *Behavioral and Brain Sciences*, **8**, pp. 567–616.

ACKNOWLEDGEMENTS

Grateful acknowledgement is made to the following sources for permission to reproduce material within this product.

Cover

Vision at end of day by Mark Rothko, National Gallery of Art, Washington;

Figures

Figure 1.2c Copyright © Douglas and Martin/Science Photo Library; *Figure 1.5* From *Neurobiology of Disease*, edited by Alan L. Pearlman, Robert C. Coli, copyright 1989 by Oxford University Press, Inc. Used by permission of Oxford University Press, Inc.; *Figures 1.6, 1.26c* and *1.29* Carpenter, R. H. S. (2002) *Neurophysiology*, 4th edition, Hodder Arnold. Copyright © R. H. S. Carpenter; *Figure 1.7b* Data from Erlanger and Gasser 1938; *Figures 1.9, 1.10, 1.14, 1.15, 1.21, 1.22a, 1.22b, 1.23* and *1.25* Kandel, E. R., Schwartz, J.H. and Jessell, T. M. (1995) *Essentials of Neural Science and Behaviour*. Copyright © 1995 The McGraw-Hill Companies, Inc; *Figure 1.11* Reprinted from *Neuron*, **31**, no 5, Schmitz, D. *et al.* 'Axo-Axonal Coupling: A novel mechanism for ultrafast neuronal communication' page 836. Copyright 2001 with permission of Elsevier; *Figure 1.13* Martini, F. H., Timmons, M. J. and McKinley, M. P. (2000) *Human Anatomy*, Prentice Hall, Upper Saddle River Inc; *Figure 1.26a and b* Brodal, A. (1981) *Neurological Anatomy in Relation to Clinical Medicine*, 3rd ed., Copyright (c) 1969, 1981, by Oxford University Press Inc. Reprinted with permission; *Figure 1.28* Kuffler, S. W., Nicholls, J. G. and Martin, A. R. (1984) *From Neuron to Brain*, 2nd edition, Sinauer Associates Inc. Publishers;

Figure 2.5 Kandel, E. R., Schwartz, J. H. and Jessell, T. M. (2000) *Principles of Neural Science*, McGraw-Hill Companies Inc.; *Figure 2.8* Gazzaniga, M. S. *et al.* 'Face cells in the superior temporal sulcus of the macaque monkey', *Prosopagnosia, Cognitive Neuroscience: The Biology of the Mind*, W. W. Norton & Co. Inc.; *Figure 2.9* Gauthier, I. *et al.* (1999) 'Activation of the middle fusiform 'face area' increases with expertise in recognising novel objects', *Nature Neuroscience*, **2**, No 6, June 1999. © Nature Publishing Group; *Figure 2.11* Kandel, E. R. 'The Bodily Senses', *Principles of Neural Science* 4th edn, Copyright © by The McGraw-Hill Companies, Inc.; *Figure 2.18* Nicholl, J. G. (2001) *From Neuron to Brain* 4th edn, Copyright 2001 Sinuaer Associates, Inc.;

Figure 3.1a From Carlson, Neil R. (2001) *Physiology Of Behavior*, 7th edn. Published by Allyn and Bacon, Boston, MA. Copyright © 2001 by Pearson Education. Reprinted by permission of the publisher; *Figure 3.1b* Carpenter, R. H. S. (2002) *Neurophysiology*, 4th edition, Hodder Arnold. Copyright © R. H. S. Carpenter; *Figures 3.2 and 3.3* Purves, D. (2001) 'A chain of nerve cells arranged in a distinhibitory circuit', *Neuroscience*, 2nd edition, Sinauer Associates Inc. *Figure 3.4a* Welker, W. 'Human homo sapiens', Brain Museum website. University of Wisconsin-Madison.

Every effort has been made to contact copyright holders. If any have been inadvertently overlooked the publishers will be pleased to make the necessary arrangements at the first opportunity.

INDEX

Glossary terms are in bold. Italics indicate items mainly, or wholly, in a figure or table.

E

ear, vestibular system, *103*, 105
Ecstasy, 37
efferent neurons *see* motor neurons
elbow, muscle movement, 64, 74, *99*, 100
electrical gradient, **3**
electrical signals, 5–13
  role of motor cortex, 92–5, 97
  role of receptors, 19–24
electrical synapses, 14–16
electricity, in the neuron, 1–5
electrodes, extracellular, 11, *12*
electromyography (EMG), 77–8
endorphins, 24
enkephalins, 24
epilepsy,
  electrical activity, 8–9
  role of motor cortex, 92
excitatory neurotransmitter, 21
excitatory postsynaptic potential (EPSP), **21**, 25–7, 65, 95
extension, 64
extensor muscles, 32, *33*
extrafusal fibres, 72, *73*
eye,
  human, 50–4
  see also vision
eye movement,
  role of basal ganglia, 90–1
  vestibular ocular reflex, 104–8

F

face recognition, 48–9, 57–60
feedback inhibition, **32**
feedback mechanism,
  multijoint movement, 102
  role of cerebellum, 108
  smooth pursuit, 105–6
feedforward inhibition, **32**, *33*
feedforward mechanism, 101–2
  in the vestibular ocular reflex, 106–8
FFA *see* fusiform face area
finger movements, 97–8, 100
  after a stroke, 99
  side to side, 104–5
firing frequency, in muscle contraction, 68
firing threshold, **7**, 8
  asynchronous firing, 67
  and neurotransmitter release, 28–30
  retinal ganglion cells, 50
flexion, 64
flexor muscles, 32, *33*, 78
FPL *see* thumb flexor muscle
Friedereich's ataxia, 103, 108
fusiform face area (FFA), **58**–60

G

GABA,
  in the brain, 36
  neurotransmission, 21, 23
  role in Huntington's disease, 38–9, 40, 88–9
  role in movement control, 91
gap junctions, **14**–16
glutamate, **23**–4
  in the brain, 36
  firing threshold, 29, *30*
  neurotransmission, 21
  removal, 22
glycine, 23
Golgi cell, *34*
grandmother, recognition, 48–9, 57, 85
'greebles', 60
Guam disease, 24

H

hand,
  motor units, 66
  muscle activation, 92, *93*, *94*, 95
  power grip, 71
  in reaching movements, 100–1, 103
  see also finger movements
head movement, side to side, 104–5
hippocampal neurons,
  effect of noradrenalin, *30*
  electrical transmission, *15*
hormones, internalization, 22
Huntington's disease, 38, 40
  function of basal ganglia, 88–9
hyperkinesis, 38
hyperpolarization, **6**–7, 8
hypokinesis, 38

I

indirectly gated ion channels, **19**–20, 21
inhibitory interneurons, 32, *33*
inhibitory postsynaptic potential (IPSP), **21**, 25, *27*, 95
intrafusal fibres, 71–2, *73*
invertebrates, electrical synapses, 14–15
ion channels, **5**–9
ions,
  action potential, 6–8
  in the neuron, 1–5
ipsilateral eye column, *53*

J

joints,
  coordination of muscle action, 75–7
  muscle movement, 64–5, 97
  position information, 73
  see also elbow; multijoint movement

K

Klippel–Feil syndrome, 82–3
knee jerk, 75, 78

L

latency of the reflex, 78–83
lateral geniculate nucleus (LGN), **52**, *53*, *54*
length–tension relationship, **70**, 71
levodopa, 37, 40
lidocaine, 9
long-latency stretch responses, 78–9, **80**, 81–3

M

magnetic resonance imaging (MRI) scanning, visual recognition, 59–60
magnocellular pathway, **52**, *53*, *54*, 55
mechanoreceptors, 49, 72, 73
membrane potential, **2**–4, 10
  permeability changes, 6–7
Mondrian display, *56*
monkeys, face recognition, 58–9
morphine, 24
mossy fibre, *34*
motor cortex, *93*
  activation, 85
  and basal ganglia, 88, 89